Intrinsic Skills for Physician Assistants

Editor

SHARONA KANOFSKY

PHYSICIAN ASSISTANT CLINICS

www.physicianassistant.theclinics.com

Consulting Editor
JAMES A. VAN RHEE

January 2020 • Volume 5 • Number 1

ELSEVIER

1600 John F. Kennedy Boulevard • Suite 1800 • Philadelphia, Pennsylvania, 19103-2899

http://www.theclinics.com

PHYSICIAN ASSISTANT CLINICS Volume 5, Number 1
January 2020 ISSN 2405-7991, ISBN-13: 978-0-323-73315-1

Editor: Katerina Heidhausen
Developmental Editor: Casey Potter

Physician Assistant Clinics (ISSN: 2405–7991) is published quarterly by Elsevier Inc., 360 Park Avenue South, New York, NY 10010-1710. Months of issue are January, April, July, and October. Periodicals postage paid at New York, NY and additional mailing offices. Subscription prices are $150.00 per year (US individuals), $216.00 (US institutions), $100.00 (US students), $150.00 (Canadian individuals), $271.00 (Canadian institutions), $100.00 (Canadian students), $150.00 (international individuals), $271.00 (international institutions), and $100.00 (international students). Foreign air speed delivery is included in all *Clinics* subscription prices. All prices are subject to change without notice. POSTMASTER: Send address changes to *Physician Assistant Clinics*, Elsevier Periodicals Customer Service, 11830 Westline Industrial Drive, St. Louis, MO 63146. Customer Service Health Sciences Division, Subscription Customer Service, 3251 Riverport Lane, Maryland Heights, MO 63043. **Customer Service: 1-800-654-2452 (U.S. and Canada); 314-447-8871 (outside U.S. and Canada). Fax: 314-447-8029. E-mail: journalscustomerservice-usa@elsevier.com (for print support); journalsonlinesupport-usa@elsevier.com (for online support).**

Reprints. For copies of 100 or more, of articles in this publication, please contact the Commercial Reprints Department, Elsevier Inc., 360 Park Avenue South, New York, NY 10010-1710. Tel. 212-633-3874; Fax: 212-633-3820; E-mail: reprints@elsevier.com.

Physician Assistant Clinics is covered in *EMBASE/Excerpta Medica and ESCI.*

PROGRAM OBJECTIVE

The goal of the *Physician Assistant Clinics* is to keep practicing physician assistants up to date with current clinical practice by providing timely articles reviewing the state of the art in patient care.

TARGET AUDIENCE

Physician Assistants and other healthcare professionals.

LEARNING OBJECTIVES

Upon completion of this activity, participants will be able to:

1. Review interprofessional communication strategies and approaches used to manage conflict scenarios and to facilitate communication among team members.
2. Discuss the value and potential pitfalls of competency-based medical education (CBME) and competency frameworks.
3. Recognize the four domains in which professionalism is demonstrated through commitment of the PA.

ACCREDITATION

The Elsevier Office of Continuing Medical Education (EOCME) is accredited by the Accreditation Council for Continuing Medical Education (ACCME) to provide continuing medical education for physicians.

The EOCME designates this journal-based CME activity for a maximum of 8 *AMA PRA Category 1 Credit*(s)™. Physicians should claim only the credit commensurate with the extent of their participation in the activity.

All other healthcare professionals requesting continuing education credit for this enduring material will be issued a certificate of participation.

DISCLOSURE OF CONFLICTS OF INTEREST

The EOCME assesses conflict of interest with its instructors, faculty, planners, and other individuals who are in a position to control the content of CME activities. All relevant conflicts of interest that are identified are thoroughly vetted by EOCME for fair balance, scientific objectivity, and patient care recommendations. EOCME is committed to providing its learners with CME activities that promote improvements or quality in healthcare and not a specific proprietary business or a commercial interest.

The planning committee, staff, authors and editors listed below have identified no financial relationships or relationships to products or devices they or their spouse/life partner have with commercial interest related to the content of this CME activity:

Esther Bennitta; Maureen Gottesman, MD, MEd, CCFP; Katerina Heidhausen; Ian W. Jones, MPAS, CCPA, PA-C; Sharona Kanofsky, PA-C, CCPA, MScCH; Alison Kemp; Sylvia Langlois, BHSc, MSc, OT Reg (ON); Dean Lising, PT, BSc, BscPT, MHSc; Casey Potter; James A. Van Rhee, MS, PA-C.

UNAPPROVED/OFF-LABEL USE DISCLOSURE

The EOCME requires CME faculty to disclose to the participants:

1. When products or procedures being discussed are off-label, unlabelled, experimental, and/or investigational (not US Food and Drug Administration [FDA] approved); and
2. Any limitations on the information presented, such as data that are preliminary or that represent ongoing research, interim analyses, and/or unsupported opinions. Faculty may discuss information about pharmaceutical agents that is outside of FDA-approved labelling. This information is intended solely for CME and is not intended to promote off-label use of these medications. If you have any questions, contact the medical affairs department of the manufacturer for the most recent prescribing information.

TO ENROLL

The CME program is available to all *Physician Assistant Clinics* subscribers at no additional fee. To subscribe to the *Physician Assistant Clinics*, call customer service at 1-800-654-2452 or sign up online at www.physicianassistant.theclinics.com.

METHOD OF PARTICIPATION

In order to claim credit, participants must complete the following:

1. Complete enrolment as indicated above.
2. Read the activity.

3. Complete the CME Test and Evaluation. Participants must achieve a score of 70% on the test. All CME Tests and Evaluations must be completed online.

CME INQUIRIES/SPECIAL NEEDS

For all CME inquiries or special needs, please contact elsevierCME@elsevier.com.

Contributors

CONSULTING EDITOR

JAMES A. VAN RHEE, MS, PA-C
Associate Professor, Program Director, Yale School of Medicine, Yale Physician Assistant Online Program, New Haven, Connecticut, USA

EDITOR

SHARONA KANOFSKY, PA-C, CCPA, MScCH
Academic Scholarship and Research Lead, Associate Professor, Teaching Stream, Physician Assistant Program, Department of Family and Community Medicine, Faculty of Medicine, University of Toronto, Toronto, Ontario, Canada

AUTHORS

MAUREEN GOTTESMAN, MD, MEd, CCFP
Assistant Professor, Department of Family and Community Medicine, Faculty of Medicine, University of Toronto, Attending Physician, Departments of Family and Community Medicine, North York General Hospital, Toronto, Ontario, Canada

IAN W. JONES, MPAS, CCPA, PA-C
Assistant Professor, Program Director, Master of Physician Assistant Studies, The University of Manitoba, Max Rady College of Medicine, Winnipeg, Manitoba, Canada

SHARONA KANOFSKY, PA-C, CCPA, MScCH
Academic Scholarship and Research Lead, Associate Professor, Teaching Stream, Physician Assistant Program, Department of Family and Community Medicine, Faculty of Medicine, University of Toronto, Toronto, Ontario, Canada

SYLVIA LANGLOIS, BHSc, MSc, OT Reg (ON)
Associate Professor, Department of Occupational Science and Occupational Therapy, Faculty Lead IPE Curriculum and Scholarship, Centre for Interprofessional Education, Faculty of Medicine, University of Toronto, University Health Network, Toronto Western Hospital, Toronto, Ontario, Canada

DEAN LISING, PT, BSc, BscPT, MHSc
Team-Based Practice and Education Lead, Director, BOOST! (Building Optimal Outcomes from Successful Teamwork) Program, IPE Scholar-in-Residence (Centennial College), Centre for Interprofessional Education, Lecturer, Department of Physical Therapy, Faculty of Medicine, University of Toronto, University Health Network, Toronto Western Hospital, Toronto, Ontario, Canada

Contents

Teaching and learning humanistic skills is a challenge. It is generally accepted that selecting for humanistic and relational character and characteristics makes the job of educators easier. Physician Assistants (PAs) must master medical knowledge, procedural skills, and humanistic competence to practice as excellent PAs.

Professionalism is a highly valued concept in the Physician Assistant (PA) profession and in all health professions. There are many definitions and descriptions of what it means to be a professional. Some of the more useful descriptions identify professionalism as both a set of values that reflect the profession, as well as a set of individual traits and characteristics that individual PAs should embody. Professionalism is shown through the commitment of the PAs in four domains: commitment to the patient, the profession, the public, and self.

Reflection is a higher-order metacognitive process that allows a Physician Assistant (PA) to identify and analyze individual challenges in practice, with the purpose of addressing these challenges. The process of reflection allows the PA to develop actionable plans to address the gaps in current knowledge, skills, or attitudes. Reflection is derived from the education psychology theories of reflective practice but has shifted from its theoretic foundations to its common use in healthcare education and practice.

Ethical decision-making in healthcare is a critical skill set that all Physician Assistants (PAs) must learn. Although PAs often are not the most responsible provider in a medical team, they should not make the mistake of thinking they are absolved of difficult decisions. The PA's involvement can have significant impact, especially when the PA has the tools to help guide the decision-making process. Having a clear and thoughtful approach for considering and resolving ethical dilemmas arising in clinical practice is an invaluable ability for any PA.

Effective communication is an intrinsic skill that is instrumental in being a practicing Physician Assistant (PA). The competencies addressed are based on a 2017 literature review on learning outcomes for communication in health professions. Why various skills are used to communicate is referred as the knowledge domain. What is being communicated is the content skills domain. How the information is communicated is the process skills domain. Internal refection and self-realization are explored in the perception skills domain. The unique role of the PA in healthcare delivery supports the relationships with communication partners in various settings and contexts.

Interprofessional team-based care is proposed as a key approach to address rising costs and increasing complexity in healthcare. Healthcare is anchored in relationships, hence the need to develop competencies to enhance interactions among team members and with patients. Interprofessional team approaches foster quality, safety, and optimal patient care. Team function is a balance of task and process. Interprofessional collaboration is not sufficient to create a high-functioning team. Additionally, barriers to collaboration are considered. Interprofessional communication strategies that enable collaborative practice, tools for managing conflict constructively, and facilitators of collaborative practice are described. Finally, collaborative leadership approaches are considered.

A qualitative approach and literature review are used to provide perspective on the paradigms and opinions on value as a key theoretic concept for Physician Assistants (PA). Considering the social implications of efficiency and effectiveness means looking at what people value, or the human factor in the PA role. The article investigates how PAs are valued in medical practice by physicians and explores the different viewpoints used in evaluating the concept of value in medicine.

Sharona Kanofsky

Competency-based medical education and competency frameworks, introduced in the 1990s, are arguably the greatest contributions to the renewal of medical education since Abraham Flexner revolutionized the field with his Flexner Report in 1910. The benefits of competency-based medical education include clear identification of learning outcomes to guide teaching and assessment; the ability to standardize curricula across jurisdictions and institutions, and establish criteria for accreditation, certification, and licensure; and the identification of interpersonal and professional skills that were previously undervalued compared with clinical knowledge and technical skills.

PHYSICIAN ASSISTANT CLINICS

SERIES OF RELATED INTEREST

Medical Clinics of North America
https://www.medical.theclinics.com/
Primary Care: Clinics in Office Practice
https://www.primarycare.theclinics.com/

THE CLINICS ARE AVAILABLE ONLINE!
Access your subscription at:
www.theclinics.com

Foreword
Intrinsic Skills

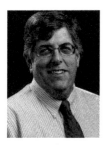

James A. Van Rhee, MS, PA-C
Consulting Editor

Intrinsic skills are those skills that come from within. We often hear these skills described as the soft side of medicine. It is the intrinsic skills that make us compassionate and caring providers. These skills are so important that the Competencies for Physician Assistant Practice devote a number of the competencies to the intrinsic skills. These include interpersonal and communication skills, professionalism, and systems-based practice.[1]

This issue of *Physician Assistant Clinics* focuses on these intrinsic skills. Sharona Kanofsky, PA-C, CCPA, MScCH, Academic Scholarship and Research Lead at the physician assistant program at the University of Toronto, has brought together a number of authors and topics that explore these intrinsic skills. Topics include professionalism for the physician assistant, reflective practice, ethical decision making, communication consideration, and collaborative working as a team.

We hope that after reading these articles the reader will reflect on how these skills impact the patients we care for, and how using these intrinsic skills, we also improve our relationship with those we work with on a daily basis. This issue should be required reading for all physician assistant students.

I hope you enjoy this issue. Our next issue will focus on Diabetes.

James A. Van Rhee, MS, PA-C
Yale School of Medicine
Yale Physician Assistant Online Program
100 Church Street South, Suite A230
New Haven, CT 06519, USA

E-mail address:
james.vanrhee@yale.edu

Website:
http://www.paonline.yale.edu

Physician Assist Clin 5 (2020) xi–xii
https://doi.org/10.1016/j.cpha.2019.09.003
2405-7991/20/© 2019 Published by Elsevier Inc.

physicianassistant.theclinics.com

REFERENCE

1. American Academy of Physician Assistants. Competencies of the PA Profession 2012. 2012. Available at: https://www.aapa.org/wp-content/uploads/2017/02/PA-Competencies-updated.pdf. Accessed September 18, 2019.

Preface
How We Use What We Know

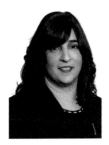

Sharona Kanofsky, PA-C, CCPA, MScCH
Editor

There is so much a physician assistant (PA) needs to know. Developing a deep and thorough knowledge of the anatomy and normal function of the human mind and body is a daunting challenge, not to mention the myriad pathologies for which patients seek our care. PAs also need to apply critical reasoning and deductive thinking processes to consider differential diagnoses, tests, referrals, and management plans. We need to remember textbooks full of information about best practice guidelines, first-line and alternate pharmacologic options, and special physical examination maneuvers to guide our assessments. Then there are the many technical and procedural skills we need to master, like suturing and central-line insertions. All this, and more, is *what* PAs need to know. But this does not address *how* we use what we know. A technically competent and knowledgeable PA does not necessarily make an excellent PA. Indeed, an excellent PA *should* strive to acquire the knowledge and technical skills, but must also possess abilities well beyond the cognitive and psychomotor.

Excellent PAs must appreciate *how* to use *what* they know. This issue addresses this constellation of abilities that is known by many names. What was once called *bedside manner* is now often referred to as *intrinsic skills*. Intrinsic skills support the medical knowledge and technical skills, allowing PAs to offer the highest-quality patient-centered care that addresses the patient's psychosocial context. The results are good health outcomes and a satisfying experience for both the patient and the PA. Essentially, intrinsic skills are relational and interpersonal. How we use our knowledge and skills in patient care depends on our ability to relate in a humanistic, caring way to our patients, our healthcare team members, and even to ourselves.

The American and Canadian PA competency frameworks highlight these intrinsic skills by identifying their respective domains. In this issue, we explore the concept of professionalism and the related processes of reflective practice and ethical decision making. We discuss the value of effective communication in gathering and conveying accurate information and in building a therapeutic PA-patient relationship. We consider

Physician Assist Clin 5 (2020) xiii–xiv
https://doi.org/10.1016/j.cpha.2019.09.002
2405-7991/20/© 2019 Published by Elsevier Inc.

how collaborative team practice in healthcare helps achieve optimal patient-centered care. We also explore the meaning of *value* in healthcare and describe how PAs enhance the value of care, from a costs-benefits perspective, but equally importantly, from the perspectives of nonmonetary value-added benefits. Finally, as the PA profession continues its global expansion, we compare the Canadian and American PA competency frameworks. We gain insight into the development of these frameworks and appreciate varying perspectives on the humanistic, relational skills that support and are inextricably linked to our clinical knowledge and procedural skills.

Sharona Kanofsky, PA-C, CCPA, MScCH
Department of Family &
Community Medicine
Faculty of Medicine
University of Toronto
263 McCaul Street, 3rd Floor
Toronto, Ontario M5T 1W7
Canada

E-mail address:
sharona.kanofsky@utoronto.ca

From Bedside Manner to Intrinsic Skills

Sharona Kanofsky, PA-C, CCPA, MScCH

KEYWORDS

- Teaching • Learning • Humanistic skills • Physician Assistant • Intrinsic skllls
- Competencies

KEY POINTS

- Teaching and learning humanistic skills is a challenge for Physician Assistant (PA) educators.
- Competence in humanistic and relational skills are as essential for PAs as competence in medical knowledge and technical expertise.
- The terminology used to describe the humanistic and relations competencies has evolved, yet there remains a consensus that they are essential components in healthcare.

INTRODUCTION

Most readers are familiar with some version of this story, either from someone they know, or from firsthand experience: a patient has a serious health concern that needs attention. A specialist consultation is required. There is a choice: there is Dr A, an expert physician who is also the leading researcher in this specialty. The only problem is that Dr A is not known for her gentle personality. She makes little eye contact, does not allow worried patients time for questions about the diagnosis or symptoms, and provides jargon-laden monologues about the prognosis and alternative treatment options that are unintelligible even to an educated lay person. Never mind her reputation in the operating room: yelling at nurses and throwing instruments around. She is a dictatorial expert; she has reviewed the patient's chart and knows exactly what she (and the patient) need to do. No questions asked. Take it or leave it. However, it is said that she has "hands of gold." She is the most technically capable expert in her field. Then there is Dr B. He has less experience than Dr A. Dr B is known as a "gem" of a person: kind, patient, attentive, and approachable. He stays with you until dawn answering all your questions and offering you alternate treatment options that match your personal preferences. Yet somehow you do not have the same degree of confidence in Dr B as you do in Dr A. Who do you go to?

Department of Family and Community Medicine, Physician Assistant Program, 263 McCaul Street, 3rd Floor, Toronto, Ontario, M5T 1W7, Canada
E-mail address: sharona.kanofsky@utoronto.ca

Physician Assist Clin 5 (2020) 1–10
https://doi.org/10.1016/j.cpha.2019.08.001
2405-7991/20/© 2019 Elsevier Inc. All rights reserved.

Of course, this is an artificially binary scenario: a caricature or a stereotype. Expertise does not have to come at the expense of kindness, caring, good communication, and a humanistic approach; nor the opposite. Competent providers should be competent in *all* areas of care: the medical knowledge and technical skills, as well as the interpersonal and relational knowledge, skills, and attitudes that make a well-rounded provider.

What society now wants from medical professionals, such as physicians and physician assistants (PAs), is competence in biomedical and clinical knowledge coupled with excellent interpersonal skills, including empathy, communication, and professionalism. This requirement is not too much to ask. A physician, or a PA, or any healthcare professional, can and should be capable in all these areas. These interpersonal skills were once referred to as a good bedside manner. Other terms have emerged in recent years, including so-called soft skills, nonmedical expert competencies, intrinsic roles, and interpersonal or relational competence.

How does a PA develop these abilities, often referred to as competencies (a set of acquired knowledge, skills, and attitudes)? For PAs, the formal training begins in PA school. All PA programs make considerable efforts to select students who already have foundational characteristics that show their ability to become excellent PAs. A high grade-point average is required, along with demonstration, in some way, of interpersonal abilities in areas such as communication and collaboration. However, the programs are themselves responsible for ensuring that the graduating PAs enter the profession with these required abilities.

Most educational programs, from grade school to higher education, focus on acquisition of knowledge. Facts are presented. The teacher's job is to convey the information; the student's job is to receive and repeat the information. Traditionally, the way educators assess whether the content has been absorbed is by having student repeat the acquired information in some verbal or written format, such as tests, essays, and other assignments. This approach works to varying degrees when the educational content is primarily academic. It is different when the educational goal is the application of knowledge and skills in some practical or professional role. The stakes are even higher when the application of this educational content is in the delivery of healthcare by health professionals. The professional abilities of a PA consequently affect the safety and well-being of patients. Simply knowing, or even mastering, the medical information or psychomotor skills to perform clinical procedures is not enough. Arguably, as much emphasis must be placed on teaching and learning medical knowledge and skills as on the abilities to appropriately apply this knowledge and skill set. PA education must be as much about application as it is about information.

WHAT VERSUS HOW

As with all healthcare professionals, PAs must be experts in their area of practice. They must learn many aspects of clinical science: the anatomy and physiology of the human body; what keeps the body and mind in a healthy state of equilibrium and what makes people sick; what are the possible diagnoses for a particular group of symptoms and which ones are most likely; what investigations to order; what is the treatment plan; and much more. All of this makes up the work of a PA, and this is the content of the PA curriculum: *what* a PA needs to know.

Just as important as the "what" aspect of PA practice, is the application of the knowledge to patient care; that is, the "how" aspects of being a PA: how you use your knowledge and content expertise to help your patients; how you listen to your patients so that they trust you and are comfortable giving you the information you need to help them; how you communicate with your patients to ensure that they understand your diagnosis and treatment plan; how you collaborate with your patients, their family members, and healthcare team members to agree on a treatment plan and ensure an optimal health outcome; how you advocate for public services available in your community; and how you provide patient education.

In short, it is not enough to know *what*, although this is vitally important. PAs needs to know *how* to use what they know to benefit patients. This "how" refers primarily to the interpersonal approach that the PA expresses at the patient encounter and in all areas of practice. Does the PA speak kindly and patiently? Does the PA listen attentively when the patient speaks? Does the PA lean in, make eye contact, convey body language and facial expressions that genuinely communicate empathy and willingness to help? Does the PA show respect and collaborate effectively with other team members?

This article explores some of the associated terms and how they came to be, and considers their merits and limitations. In each case, the terminology attempts to represent, in some way and with varying degrees of success, how health professional use what they know in the care of patients.

SOFT SKILLS

The designation of interpersonal abilities as soft skills compared with the so-called hard skills of clinical scientific knowledge and psychomotor abilities can be misleading. It suggests that these skills are easier to acquire or, worse, that they are less important in the patient's overall care experiences and health outcomes. Neither of these is true. There is nothing soft or secondary about these abilities. Although the medical knowledge and skill of PAs are central to their expertise, they cannot stand on their own. A PA with a mastery of medical skills and knowledge may still not be a capable PA without competence in areas such as communication, professionalism, teamwork, and advocacy. Although PA education typically aspires to teach the knowledge, skills, and attitudes required of PAs, of these three domains, attitudes can be the most difficult to teach, learn, demonstrate and assess. The relational skills of clinicians have been shown to have a significant impact on multiple measures of health outcomes, including satisfaction,[1,2] compliance,[3] safety,[4] and health outcomes.[5,6]

In *The Good Doctor in Medical Education 1910–2010: a Critical Discourse Analysis*, Cynthia Whitehead[7] describes the evolution of what it has meant to be a good doctor at different times over roughly the last century, in relation to shifting social factors, such as economics and public values. Although PAs are not the focus of her analysis, this article suggests that much of what applies to the ideals of a good doctor can also apply to the conceptualization of a good PA. Although the history and development of the PA and physician professions differ significantly, both professions value interpersonal competencies, and the similarities and overlapping themes are useful to consider.

The year 1910 was a major landmark, often considered the start of modern medical education. The central figure of this shift was a doctor named Abraham Flexner, who authored the famous Flexner Report on medical education in Canada and the United States, commissioned by the Carnegie Foundation.[8] He described the ideal physician as a scientist and a well-rounded, educated gentleman. Before this time, medical schools varied greatly in their admissions and education standards. Some were private commercial schools of varying quality, which Flexner looked on disdainfully, attributing to these schools "a century of reckless over-production of cheap doctors."[8(p15)] Among his many accomplishments in this area, Flexner helped standardize the admissions process and curricular content, emphasizing biomedical sciences, and rigorous admissions and academic standards. Flexner's view was that a good physician practices by applying a solid foundation of scientific knowledge and by behaving in a distinguished, gentlemanly manner. This scientific foundation of medicine may seem obvious now, but it was not obvious at the time, when much of medical practice was based on often subjective observations, empirical evidence, untested theory, and even superstitious beliefs. Although the Flexnerian physician was compared with a master craftsman, the old apprenticeship model of medical learning was rejected. "The place and the way to train his master craftsman scientist are within the hallowed halls of academe, not out on the dirt roads or homes of the sick."[7(p60)]

Although Flexner's renewal of medical education was cutting edge at the time, many of his views are at once quaint, but antiquated. For one, physicians of the time were expected to be *gentlemen* of social stature; a female physician was unthinkable. However, the relationship with the patient remained a priority. Flexner considered with fondness the bedside opportunities afforded by the apprenticeship model of medical training. A romantic image of this educational model conjures the apprentice and his master riding through the countryside by horse and buggy, to the homes and bedsides of sick patients. Despite his emphasis on standardized medical education, Flexner approved of this form of clinical bedside learning.

BEDSIDE MANNER

The term bedside manner is an old, generalized expression that refers to the attitude, disposition, and interaction that a healthcare provider displays to a patient. This concept includes a variety of unspecified verbal and nonverbal expressions of care, empathy, and effective communication skills. The term implies that patient care, to a significant degree, occurs in proximity to, and in communication with, the patient. The presence or absence of an effective bedside manner is traditionally a judgment made by the patient based on the healthcare professional's interpersonal abilities. Patient satisfaction and compliance are usually linked to a judgment of the care provider's bedside manner. The term bedside manner is not used in objective assessments of medical trainees' abilities. The concept of bedside manner aligns with Flexner's ideals and with the notion of the good PA as a person of character.

Bedside manner may sound dated, but it also takes on new meaning in the current age of high-speed healthcare, in which clinicians have only a few minutes to interact with each patient directly, at the bedside. This limitation is true across all healthcare settings, from inpatient hospital care to the emergency department; from the family or walk-in clinic to the operating room.

During the author's coursework toward a master's in health professions education, many of her classmates were young family physicians. They frequently lamented that one of their biggest challenges is the disappointment of the imposed time pressure in practice, resulting in not enough time to spend with their patients; not having time to get to know their patients or to address all their issues, as they had imagined during their training. "This is not what I went to medical school for," was a common complaint against the imposed pressures of clinical practice. However, one of the things PAs consistently report about their own practice is the ability to spend more time with patients, compared with physicians.[9] In this way, PAs can perhaps have a greater impact in preventive care and effective patient education.

BEDSIDE AND TECHNOLOGY

Just as household appliances were exalted as time-saving devices that would provide homemakers of the early twentieth century with more leisure time, computers in healthcare are purported to free clinicians to spend more time at the bedside. The irony that electronic charting, documentation, and ordering of tests seem to produce the opposite effect is lost on few healthcare professionals.[10] Paradoxically, the decreasing time available for patient interactions seems to mirror the high speed of these technological advances. The tasks that prevent clinicians from spending more time with their patients include the constant need to use computers in patient care: to update the patient chart with the latest clinical notes; retrieve patient information, such as recent laboratory data; look up updated evidence-based care guidelines and best practices for specific clinical scenarios; or search and print appropriate patient education literature to help the patients understand their conditions. These uses of computers and the Internet are all valuable and appropriate, but they take away from the dwindling and precious resource of time at the bedside.

There are two approaches to this conundrum, both of which can be attempted simultaneously. One is embedded in the term bedside manner. It is simply to make a concerted effort to stay at the bedside of the patient by learning to value this as time well spent. It has become an almost involuntary reflex to spend the minimum time at the bedside. There are many reasons for this embedded in the so-called hidden curriculum of medical culture. Clinicians tend to do as they see others doing in the clinical setting, despite what they may have learned to value or what they have learned in the classroom. One small intervention that could have a big impact on medical and PA education, could simply be teaching trainees how to sit. It has been shown that simply sitting at the bedside of a patient, rather than standing, can significantly increase patient satisfaction, therapeutic rapport, and patient compliance with management plans. These factors, in turn, are all predictors of positive health outcomes, decreased lengths of hospital stay, decreased costs, and decreased litigation.[11]

The second thing that can be done, because computer use is not optional, is to include the computer in the bedside patient encounter. This strategy is already in place in many hospitals and clinics, and should be implemented everywhere, as best practice. Rather than charting and searching for information at a designated station away from the patient, this work can be done at the bedside, with patient engagement and involvement. For example, while searching for patient educational literature online, PAs could include the patient in the search. Just as PAs already know how to multitask (eg, by continuing gathering health history information or providing patient education while performing a physical examination), PAs can also continue their conversations with patients while looking together at the screen and thinking aloud about their care. A deliberate use of technology, even strategically positioning the computer screen at the bedside to avoid having the PA's back to the patient, can prevent computer use from disrupting bedside care.

THE GROWTH OF CHARACTERISTICS

The early part of the twentieth century gave rise to a new era of psychological analysis and psychometrics. Although Flexner's[7] ideals of good character were still in focus, there began a shift to measuring characteristics, rather than character, in medical education and practice.[7(pp127–75)] Medical school applicants were subject to a barrage of testing, including tests of intelligence, aptitude, interests, and even psychological stability. By the 1960s, the emphasis of medical admissions and practice had fully shifted from viewing physicians as whole people (ie, character) to being a sum of multiple parts (ie, characteristics). From this shift in focus from character to characteristics, it is possible to extrapolate a line to the current situation in health sciences education and practice; namely, to emphasizing outcomes and competencies, as described by the various roles-based competency frameworks, such as the Accreditation Council for Graduate Medical Education (ACGME) Core Competencies[12] and CanMEDS for physicians[13], and CanMEDS-PA[14] and American Academy of PAs (AAPA) Competencies for the Physician Assistant Profession.[15]

ROLES ROLL IN

The profession of medicine reached a peak of social stature and authority in the 1950s and 1960s. However, by the 1970s, medicine came under increasing social scrutiny and began losing some of its autonomy. Some of the contributing factors were increasing size and complexity of healthcare systems around the world, causing centralizing of administration and resource management; increasing access to medical knowledge, causing a decline in the authority and ownership of medicine's expertise; and increasing healthcare costs, leading to increased scrutiny about physician compensation and social demands for accountability. For example, physicians went on strike in Ontario in 1986 over the practice of so-called extra billing, whereby physicians would charge patients more than the fees that the government had set for medical services. Physicians thought that their services were not being compensated adequately. They also believed themselves threatened by the loss of autonomy in setting their own fees. Doctors were surprised that the public did not support the strike; instead, the physician community's reputation was tarnished, and the strike resulted in a blow to physicians' public image.[16]

Along with the public demands for professional accountability came renewed calls for standardization in medical education and practice. The phenomenon, famously labeled "the death of expertise" by Thomas Nichols[17] in his book of that title, emerged across the professions. Physicians started wondering what the public thought a good physician should be. Physician expertise and behavior began to take shape using the language of outcomes, performance, and competencies. Rather than asking about characteristics, the questions turned to what a physician should be able to do? What skills can a competent physician perform? In what specific knowledge, skills, attitudes, or behaviors should a physician be competent? These areas of competence needed to be organized and categorized in order to be taught, learned, and assessed at the curricular, accreditation, and continuing professional development levels. In order to categorize these newly identified areas of competence, competency frameworks emerged (in some frameworks, they are called roles, whereas in others they are referred to as domains. This distinction is considered in the article comparing the Canadian and American competency frameworks elsewhere in this issue).

Early examples of competency frameworks included the ACGME framework in the United States and The Royal College of Physicians and Surgeons of Canada (RCPSC) framework in Canada, both projects initially designed for graduate medical training. The ACGME's Outcomes Project identified six general competency domains: patient care, medical knowledge, practice-based learning and improvement, interpersonal and communication skills, professionalism, and systems-based practice.[18] The RCPSC's CanMEDS framework identified 7 roles: medical expert, communicator, collaborator, manager, health advocate, scholar, and professional.[13] These roles were subsequently updated, and the role of leader has now replaced manager.[14]

For PAs, the AAPA competency framework domains are: patient-centered practice knowledge, society and population health, health literacy and communication, interprofessional collaborative practice and leadership, professional and legal aspects of healthcare, and healthcare finance and systems.[15] The Canadian Association of Physician Assistants competency framework for PAs, CanMEDS-PA, has mirrored much of the language of CanMEDS, the framework on which it is modeled, including updating the manager role to leader in the latest iteration updated in 2015.

Other professional and educational bodies have also adopted and adapted the CanMEDS framework. Examples include the professional competency profiles for the physiotherapy and the occupation therapy professions in Canada,[19,20] and the framework for undergraduate medical education in the Netherlands.[21]

NONMEDICAL EXPERT ROLES

At some time after the development of the CanMEDS competency framework in Canada, the interpersonal roles acquired the spurious shorthand nickname of nonmedical expert roles. The RCPSC's CanMEDS framework (See Fig. 1 in "Competency-Based Medical Education for Physician Assistants: The Development of Competency-Based Medical Education and Competency Frameworks in the United States and Canada" in this issue) is represented as a venn diagram that has been noted to resemble a flower. The Medical Expert Role is central in the diagram, representing the centrality of this role for medical professionals. The other supporting roles are situated peripherally, resembling petals of a flower. All of the roles overlap with each other, representing the interrelatedness and interdependence of all areas of competence.

This visual representation inadvertently gave rise to a critical view of the supporting roles as secondary in status in the development of medical professionals. If these roles are secondary and subservient to the Medical Expert Role, by implication, they are also less important, and perhaps even nonessential. This criticism stood in sharp contrast to the stated purpose of the roles-based framework, which was to name the various roles, and thereby to increase them in prominence; to identify specific and (ideally) measurable educational outcomes. It was even speculated that these so-called nonmedical expert roles were a defensive reaction by the medical profession to social threats to its authority and autonomy. While the RCPSC never considered the diagram to represent a flower, nevertheless, this resemblance provoked the criticism. It was suggested that, the petals were intended to act as armour, surrounding and thereby protecting the medical expertise of physicians.[22,23]

Another important criticism of the roles frameworks is that separating the roles into distinct components, and fragmenting the outcomes into checklist items, would result in an overemphasis on the granular details, while losing sight of the bigger picture, the whole being more than the sum of its parts.

INTRINSIC ROLES

In response to this criticism of the roles and outcomes model, some of the original developers of the CanMEDS framework suggested a shift, from what they called the pejorative term nonmedical expert roles, to the term intrinsic roles.[24] They asserted that the term nonmedical expert roles was never used in the development of CanMEDS, and that, essentially, it is a rogue term that emerged in the educational and clinical settings. They argued that the "proposed change in nomenclature will situate the Intrinsic Roles not as appendages, add-ons, or politically-defensive armour, but as intrinsic (i.e. inherent, fundamental, essential) to the practice of medicine, integrated with each other and the Medical Expert Role."[24(p696)] The term intrinsic roles has since become the correct operational term for the supporting roles (the roles surrounding the central Medical Expert Role) sanctioned by the CanMEDS framework. It sounds better than nonmedical expert roles and promotes the importance of these roles. However, it does not completely capture their essence.

INTERPERSONAL OR RELATIONAL COMPETENCE

Although the term intrinsic roles promotes the validity of these competency domains, by designating them as "inherent, fundamental, essential,"[24(p696)] it does not quite describe their nature. What are the essential qualities of the intrinsic roles? In attempting to shed light on this question, it may be useful to look at the feedback that originally led to the development of CanMEDS, one of the most well-known and successful of the competency frameworks. The development of the CanMEDS framework followed, and picked up, where the Educating Future Physicians of Ontario (EFPO) project left off. The EFPO project was a collaboration between the five medical schools in Ontario in the early 1990s. The purpose was to renew medical education curricula to align with societal views of what physician roles should be. Following extensive surveys of stakeholders and the public, it was determined that one of the desired or expected roles was that of humanist. This role was based on the frequent feedback that identified the ideal physician as more than a medical expert and a gatekeeper to medical services; a physician should also possess interpersonal and relational skills in order to interact well with patients at an individual level.[7(p176)]

Many of the current intrinsic roles emerged from this initial humanist prototype role. It is perhaps fitting to revisit this original intention and call these intrinsic roles what they really are: interpersonal or relational competence. This descriptive terminology is both more appealing and more accurate, based on what was described earlier in the development of this framework.

As an added point, during a time when technological advances encroach on the personal aspects of healthcare delivery, it is possibly even more important to emphasize the human, the humane, the interpersonal, and the relational aspects of healthcare. As machines, computers, and robots become capable of doing some of the work of people, often and increasingly better than people, these interpersonal and relational skills are perhaps one of the few things that humans will still do better than machines (at least for the near future).

SUMMARY

This article discusses the relational abilities that emphasize the humane, caring, and compassionate aspects of healthcare. It argues that these abilities are at least equally important to cognitive and psychomotor abilities. These abilities are important, even central, to PA practice. Excellence in knowledge and skills is the sine qua non of PA practice. However, the relational and interpersonal skills are what distinguish PAs from mere technicians and, arguably, what set PAs apart from machines who can store more information and perform more accurate technical procedures.

Calling the intrinsic roles what they are - interpersonal or relational competencies - brings the discussion back to where it began. How PAs practice medicine and care for patients is at least as important as what they know.

Teaching and learning humanistic skills is a challenge. Admissions and selections committees try to crack this code perennially. It is generally accepted that selecting for humanistic and relational character and characteristics makes the job of educators easier. However, much of this education will still be the job of PA educators, to ensure

PAs enter the profession with at least as much of this skill set with which they entered the PA program and, it is hoped, much more.

Whether it is called bedside manner, intrinsic skills, interpersonal or relational competencies, the conclusion remains: PAs must develop the medical knowledge, procedural skills, and humanistic competence to practice as excellent PAs.

ACKNOWLEDGMENTS

The author would like to thank the Consortium of PA Education, the Department of Family & Community Medicine, and the University of Toronto for supporting the preparation of this article.

REFERENCES

1. Clark PAMPA. Medical practices' sensitivity to patients' needs: opportunities and practices for improvement. J Ambul Care Manage 2003;26(2):110–23. Available at: https://ovidsp.ovid.com/ovidweb.cgi?T=JS&CSC=Y&NEWS=N&PAGE=fulltext&D=ovftf&AN=00004479-200304000-00004.
2. Wanzer MB, Booth-Butterfield M, Gruber K. Perceptions of Health Care Providers' Communication: Relationships Between Patient-Centered Communication and Satisfaction. Health Commun 2004;16(3):363–84. Available at: http://resolver.scholarsportal.info/resolve/10410236/v16i0003/363_pohcpcrbpcas.
3. Heisler M, Bouknight RR, Hayward RA, et al. The relative importance of physician communication, participatory decision making, and patient understanding in diabetes self-management. J Gen Intern Med 2002;17(4):243–52. Available at: https://www.ncbi.nlm.nih.gov/pubmed/11972720 https://www.ncbi.nlm.nih.gov/pmc/PMC1495033/.
4. Leonard M, Graham S, Bonacum D. The human factor: the critical importance of effective teamwork and communication in providing safe care. Qual Saf Healthc 2004;13(Suppl 1):i85–90.
5. Stewart M, Brown JB, Donner A, et al. The impact of patient-centered care on outcomes. J Fam Pract 2000;49(9):796–804.
6. Stewart MA. Effective physician-patient communication and health outcomes: a review. CMAJ 1995;152(9):1423–33. Available at: https://www.ncbi.nlm.nih.gov/pubmed/7728691 https://www.ncbi.nlm.nih.gov/pmc/PMC1337906/.
7. Whitehead C. The good doctor in medical education 1910–2010: a critical discourse analysis. Ann Arbor (MI): University of Toronto (Canada); 2011. Available at: https://search-proquest-com.myaccess.library.utoronto.ca/docview/1325198992#. Dissertations & Theses @ University of Toronto; ProQuest Dissertations & Theses Global database. (NR79370).
8. Flexner A. Medical education in the United States and Canada. From the Carnegie Foundation for the Advancement of Teaching, Bulletin Number Four, 1910. Bulletin of the World Health Organization 2002;80(7):594–602.
9. Timmermans MJ, van Vught AJ, Van den Berg M, et al. Physician Assistants in Medical Ward Care: A Descriptive Study of the Situation in the Netherlands. J Eval Clin Pract 2016;22(3):395–402.
10. Gawande A. The upgrade. The New Yorker 2018;94(36):62. Available at: http://link.galegroup.com/apps/doc/A561594809/BIC?u=utoronto_main&sid=BIC&xid=1de176e9.
11. Swayden KJ, Anderson KK, Connelly LM, et al. Effect of sitting vs. standing on perception of provider time at bedside: A pilot study. Patient Educ Couns

2012;86(2):166–71. Available at: http://resolver.scholarsportal.info/resolve/07383991/v86i0002/166_eosvsotabaps.

12. Holmboe ES, Laura E, Stan H. The Milestones Guidebook. Chicago: Accreditation Council for Graduate Medical Education; 2016.

13. Frank JR, Danoff D. The CanMEDS initiative: implementing an outcomes-based framework of physician competencies. Med Teach 2007;29(7):642–7. Available at: http://resolver.scholarsportal.info/resolve/0142159x/v29i0007/642_tciiaofopc.

14. CanMEDS: Better standards, better physicians, better care. CanMEDS Framework. Available at: http://www.royalcollege.ca/rcsite/canmeds/canmeds-framework-e. Accessed August 5, 2019.

15. Competencies for the Physician Assistant Profession. National Commission on Certification of Physician Assistants; 2012. Available at: https://prodcmsstoragesa.blob.core.windows.net/uploads/files/PACompetencies.pdf. Accessed October 16, 2019.

16. Butt H, Jacalyn D. Educating Future Physicians for Ontario and the Physicians' Strike of 1986: The Roots of Canadian Competency-Based Medical Education. Canadian Medical Association journal 2018;190(7):E196–8.

17. Nichols TM. The death of expertise: the campaign against established knowledge and why it matters. New York: Oxford University Press, Inc; 2017.

18. Swing SR. The ACGME outcome project: retrospective and prospective. Med Teach 2007;29(7):648–54. Available at: http://resolver.scholarsportal.info/resolve/0142159x/v29i0007/648_taoprap.

19. Essential competencies of practice for occupational therapists in Canada. 3rd edition. Association of Canadian Occupational Therapy Regulatory Organizations; 2011. Available at: https://www.coto.org/docs/default-source/essential-competencies/3rd-essential-competencies_ii_may-2011.pdf?sfvrsn=2.

20. Essential competency profile for physiotherapists in Canada. National Physiotherapy Advocacy Group; 2009. Available at: http://www.physiotherapy education.ca/Resources/Essential%20Comp%20PT%20Profile%202009.pdf.

21. Laan RF, Leunissen RR, van Herwaarden CL. The 2009 framework for undergraduate medical education in the Netherlands. GMS Z Med Ausbild 2010;27(2): Doc35. Available at: https://www.ncbi.nlm.nih.gov/pubmed/21818204 https://www.ncbi.nlm.nih.gov/pmc/articles/PMC3140367/.

22. Whitehead C, Austin Z, Hodges B. Flower power: the armoured expert in the CanMEDS competency framework? Adv Health Sci Educ Theory Pract 2011;16(5): 681–94. Available at: http://resolver.scholarsportal.info/resolve/13824996/v16i0005/681_fptaeitccf.

23. Berwick DM, Nolan TW, Whittington J. The triple aim: care, health, and cost. Health Aff (Millwood) 2008;27(3):759–69. Available at: http://myaccess.library.utoronto.ca/login?url=https://search.proquest.com/docview/204518979?accountid=14771 http://partneraccess.oclc.org/wcpa/servlet/Search?wcapi=1&wcpartner=proquesta&wcautho=100-167-144&wcissn=02782715&wcdoctype=ser.

24. Sherbino J, Frank J, Flynn L, et al. "Intrinsic Roles" rather than "armour": renaming the "non-medical expert roles" of the CanMEDS framework to match their intent. Adv Health Sci Educ Theory Pract 2011;16(5):695–7. Available at: http://resolver.scholarsportal.info/resolve/13824996/v16i0005/695_rrtrtecftmti https://link.springer.com/article/10.1007%2Fs10459-011-9318-z.

Professionalism for Physician Assistants

Sharona Kanofsky, PA-C, CCPA, MScCH

KEYWORDS

- Professionalism • Physician Assistant • Health professions • Ethics • Medicine

KEY POINTS

- Professionalism is a highly valued concept in the physician assistant (PA) profession and in all health professions. There are many definitions and descriptions of what it means to be a professional.
- Some of the more useful descriptions identify professionalism as both a set of values that reflect the profession, as well as a set of individual traits and characteristics that individual PAs should embody.
- Professionalism is demonstrated through the PA's commitment in four domains: commitment to the patient, the profession, the public, and self.

INTRODUCTION

A student recently asked me, "Why is there so much talk about professionalism? Doesn't it basically mean doing your job well, treating everyone respectfully, dressing appropriately, and showing up on time?" She has a point. A lot has been written in efforts to define professionalism and describe what it means to be a professional. So why are these such difficult questions? Although knowledge of health and disease is more clear-cut, professionalism is challenging to define and pin down. Clinicians can point to a broken bone or a diseased lung on a radiograph, but professionalism seems more elusive and abstract. However, clinicians have a deep sense that it is an important and indispensable component of healthcare practice. This article examines these concepts to gain a better understanding of this complex topic.

Professionalism, although challenging to define, can be partially, but not completely, identified by a set of attitudes and behaviors. These elements can vary from one definition to another. Because of this variation, and because of its complex nature, professionalism cannot be defined only as a set of identifiable characteristics.

To better understand professionalism, this article also explores the domains in which it is expressed. Physician Assistants (PAs) demonstrate professionalism

Faculty of Medicine, Department of Family and Community Medicine, Physician Assistant Program, 263 McCaul Street, 3rd Floor, Toronto, Ontario, M5T 1W7, Canada
E-mail address: sharona.kanofsky@utoronto.ca

Physician Assist Clin 5 (2020) 11–26
https://doi.org/10.1016/j.cpha.2019.08.002
2405-7991/20/© 2019 Elsevier Inc. All rights reserved.
physicianassistant.theclinics.com

through a commitment to the following domains: the patient, the public, the PA profession, and self.

Professionalism is also closely linked to the word profession. This article considers the nature of professions and how this relates to the notion of professionalism. The focus is on what these terms mean specifically in the context of the PA profession.

In addition, this article considers some of the specific characteristics associated with professionalism, to gain a deeper understanding of what they mean in the context of PA practice, how these terms may be helpful, and what challenges they may present.

WHAT IS PROFESSIONALISM?

The Canadian competency framework for PAs, CanMEDS-PA,[1(p21)] defines the role of the professional as a commitment "to the health and well-being of individuals and society through ethical practice, profession-led association, and high personal standards of behavior." It further elaborates that, "The professional role is guided by a code of ethics and commitment to clinical competence, embracing the appropriate attitudes and behaviors, integrity, altruism, personal wellbeing and the promotion of public good within their scope of practice."[1(p21)] The elements of professionalism are further elaborated and categorized within four specific domains: commitment to patient, commitment to society, commitment to the profession, and commitment to self.[1]

The American Competencies for the Physician Assistant Profession address similar themes, with some differences. They describe professionalism as "the expression of positive values and ideals as care is delivered. Foremost, it involves prioritizing the interests of those being served above one's own. Physician Assistants must acknowledge their professional and personal limitations. Professionalism also requires that PAs practice without impairment from substance abuse, cognitive deficiency or mental illness. Physician Assistants must demonstrate a high level of responsibility, ethical practice, sensitivity to a diverse patient population, and adherence to legal and regulatory requirements."[2]

The American framework goes on to list several specific expectations that reflect professionalism, including understanding the role and laws related to PA practice; establishing professional relationships with others in the team; showing professional traits and behaviors, such as respect, compassion, integrity, accountability, sensitivity to diversity, self-care, and reflection; and commitment to excellence and ethical practice.[2]

Between the American and Canadian PA descriptions of professionalism described above, most of the key features of professionalism can be found that are common to other descriptions and definitions of professionalism that are encountered. These definitions include commitment to the health of patients and populations; ethical practice and high moral standards; professional organization; and so-called appropriate attitudes and behaviors, such as altruism and self-care. In these two frameworks, the characterization of professionalism is also encountered as a set of general attitudes and values as well as a collection of specific behaviors and personal characteristics. Professionalism is, at once, both an overarching value system and a group of identifiable behaviors and traits.

The origin of the word profession dates to the twelfth century and relates to a "declaration, promise, or vow made by a person entering a religious order."[3] Later, it came to represent any solemn declaration, or vow, not necessarily religious. Consider then, that when people enter the PA profession, they take on a solemn commitment. This commitment elevates their work beyond a mere series of duties and tasks. Many people describe their own path to the health professions as a calling or a duty to care for others. Entering the PA profession includes measures of commitment, altruism, and a willingness to go beyond the usual demands of a job. There is a general consensus that a profession is more than a job, and that caring for humans and their well-being is a sacred duty that goes beyond merely earning a livelihood.

Like the American and Canadian descriptions of the professionalism domain/role in the respective competency frameworks, most definitions of the terms profession and professionalism highlight common features. Typically, a definition of profession includes mastery of a highly specialized body of knowledge that is studied rigorously in an academic setting. Once applied in practice, and with experience gained over time, professionals become experts in the profession. This specialized body of knowledge and abilities is typically not readily accessible to the lay public, who use, and benefit from, the services of the profession. The ownership of this specialized body of knowledge and abilities by the profession assumes a responsibility to use these abilities ethically and for the benefit of the public. Belonging to a profession often implies a privileged position in society and the right to self-regulate. It also assumes a degree of public entrustment of the expertise to the profession, and the belief in the good will of professionals to use their expertise for the benefit of society.

Cruess and colleagues[4] offer a working definition for profession, which was used to develop the Royal College of Physicians and Surgeons of Canada's CanMEDS description of the professional role, which, in turn, informed the CanMEDS-PA description of the same role:

> *Profession: An occupation whose core element is work based upon the mastery of a complex body of knowledge and skills. It is a vocation in which knowledge of some department of science or learning or the practice of an art founded upon it is used in the service of others. Its members are governed by codes of ethics and profess a commitment to competence, integrity and morality, altruism, and the promotion of the public good within their domain. These commitments form the basis of a social contract between a profession and society, which in return grants the profession a monopoly over the use of its knowledge base, the right to considerable autonomy in practice and the privilege of self-regulation. Professions and their members are accountable to those served and to society.[4(p75)]*

This definition includes the features discussed previously. A profession represents ownership of a complex body of knowledge and skills; service to the public is a key attribute of professionalism, underpinned by an assumed social contract; and members of the profession are guided by a code of ethics and altruistic characteristics.

CanMEDS-PA identifies the domains of professional behavior by describing the PA's commitment to patients, society, the profession, and self. This article examines each of these domains in turn.

COMMITMENT TO THE PATIENT

Commitment to patients demands excellence in clinical practice and maintaining competence in the knowledge, skills, and attitudes of PA practice, all while following the values of the profession, such as those outlined in the Canadian PA code of ethics.[5] Excellence in practice begins with a solid educational foundation, provided in an accredited PA training program, and continues with lifelong habits of reflective practice, self-directed learning, and professional development. Commitment to patients also means providing compassionate and conscientious care, and prioritizing the patient's well-being, but not at the expense of the PA's own personal well-being, as discussed later. This commitment is what PAs solemnly profess to do when they enter the profession. In whatever professional activities they engage, their patients must always be the center of their focus. This requirement may be obvious when interviewing a patient or standing at the bedside performing a clinical procedure. It may not be as obvious when attending a medical conference, lobbying at a state or provincial assembly, or maintaining certification by logging continuing professional development hours. However, on brief reconsideration of these professional activities, it requires minimal imagination to recognize that patients are also at the center of each one. When clinicians engage in professional development for themselves, they become better PAs for their patients. Patient-centered care requires PAs to prioritize the well-being of the patients and to consider the patients in all professional activities, whether in direct contact with the patients or otherwise.

COMMITMENT TO THE PUBLIC

As mentioned previously, professionalism reaches beyond a list of appropriate behaviors and attitudes shown in patient interactions. Some clinicians have suggested that professionalism should also be viewed through a sociologic lens, accounting for societal, historical, and even institutional contexts. Several sociologic approaches to professionalism in medical education literature are identified by Martimianakis and colleagues,[6] including professionalism as a role played in society, as a social construct, and as a means of social control. These approaches relate specifically to the profession of medicine with its so-called dominant social position.[7] However, these approaches should also be considered as they relate to the PA profession. For example, professionalism as a role in society implies that an individual professional's behavior is a reflection on the profession, which, in turn, functions as a service to society. This point is especially true in the context of a new and emerging profession, such as the PA profession in non-US countries, and even in the United States, to some extent. Each PA is proportionally more representative of the profession than individuals in more highly populated professions, such as medicine and nursing.

As a PA, commitment to society requires a proficient understanding of the healthcare system and of the social determinants of health. PAs should understand the structures and functions of the healthcare systems in which they work, and appreciate how their profession is situated within these systems. PAs may function differently in different settings and it is the PAs' responsibility to understand how they will function within the specific context in which they work.

Commitment to society further requires an understanding of the special status granted to health professionals within society. PAs, like physicians, nurses, and other health professionals, have a specialized body of knowledge and abilities. This specialized status comes with a set of responsibilities and privileges, often referred to as a social contract. The term social contract was first used to describe the relationship between citizens and their rulers or governors. The concept suggests a reciprocal relationship of rights and privileges on both sides. The term later came to be used in the medical profession when professionalism, in general, was increasing.[8] The elements of this social contract are described in the literature as follows: "Society's expectations of medicine are: the services of the healer, assured competence, altruistic service, morality and integrity, accountability, transparency, objective advice, and promotion of the public good. Medicine's expectations of society are: trust, autonomy, self-regulation, a healthcare system that is value-driven and adequately funded, participation in public policy, shared responsibility for health, a monopoly, and both non-financial and financial rewards."[9(p170)]

The lay person does not have the same access to the specialized areas of knowledge and abilities, and therefore cannot fully evaluate the services received from a professional. Patients and society may be able to express satisfaction or appreciate a general sense of quality, but much of the service is received based on the public's trust that PAs possess the abilities to which they profess. PAs' trustworthy service to society elevates their work and their public service; it is not merely a business, a job, or a livelihood. They must also recognize the power differential that is created in this trusting relationship and strive to provide the type of excellent care that justifies this trust. PAs' may also use their privileged position to enhance their personal lives by achieving an acceptable work-life balance, experiencing satisfaction in their work, and even by earning a respectable salary doing it, but this must be done in a way that balances their own needs with the best interest of the patient and society.

These elements of the social contract, described by Cruess and colleagues,[4] seem incomplete or partly outdated. For example, suggesting that the social contract "grants the profession a monopoly over the use of its knowledge base,"[4(p75)] may be an overstatement in an era when many professions overlap in scope, and when medical information is easily accessible to the public. When considering physicians and PAs, the knowledge base overlaps, and physicians cannot claim a monopoly over this content. Furthermore, the "privilege of self-regulation,"[4(p74)] does not necessarily apply to all professions. For example, PAs are currently not regulated in Ontario, which raises the question of whether regulation is indeed a requirement to be considered a profession.

COMMITMENT TO THE PHYSICIAN ASSISTANT PROFESSION

The whole is greater than the sum of the parts. This saying can describe the power of collective commitment to a person's own profession and professional organizations. Commitment and accountability to the profession goes hand in hand with commitment to the patients and to the public. There are many ways to do this, some involving greater investment than others. At the more accessible end of the investment scale, at a minimum, all PAs should join their professional organization as members. In addition to the larger national organizations, such as the American Academy for PAs (AAPA) and the Canadian Association of Physician Assistants (CAPA), there are also opportunities to join constitutional organizations, such as state chapters and specialty associations. For PAs who have the inclination and abilities, there are many opportunities to get involved in professional organizations and show a commitment to the PA profession.

Especially in a small and growing profession such as the PA profession in Canada, each individual PA represents the profession disproportionately, compared with other larger professions. PAs in countries where the profession is just emerging are establishing their role in the healthcare system; first impressions are often lasting. By elevating themselves as PAs to the highest ideals of their profession, they can, in a very real way, elevate the entire profession. Responsibility to the profession includes accountability to related laws, policies, and regulatory bodies; commitment to patient safety and quality improvement; managing conflicts of interest in the workplace; and a commitment to the professional code of ethics.[1]

The College of Family Physicians of Canada suggest three levels at which to practice social accountability. These opportunities exist at the micro, meso, and macro levels, represented as a set of expanding concentric circles.[10–13] The micro level takes place in the clinical environment, in the relationships with patients and interactions with the interprofessional team.[11] The meso level encompasses the local community and geographic region where the clinician works.[13] The macro level includes involvement in health policies and public health issues.[12] This model can be borrowed to describe different levels of opportunity for PAs to show commitment to the profession.

At the micro level, PAs can promote the profession in daily interpersonal interactions. PAs can educate patients and healthcare team members about their professional role, or promote the profession by providing excellent care and by working effectively within the healthcare team. At the meso level, PAs can be involved in local health initiatives or take on teaching roles in PA education, such as supervising students in clinical placements. At the macro level, PAs can advocate for laws that support PA practice or meet with local elected officials to advance public health policy initiatives.

COMMITMENT TO SELF

Caring for sick patients is highly demanding and often stressful work. PAs must care for themselves in order to be able to provide high-quality care for their patients and avoid the potential pitfalls of occupational burnout. At the most basic level, PAs must care for themselves by acquiring healthy habits, such as healthy eating, physical activity, adequate rest, and leisure. They should access their own health services, addressing physical or mental health issues when they arise. To help promote holistic wellness, they should consider mindfulness and meditative practices. PAs should also avoid harmful behaviors, such as substance or alcohol misuse. Caring for self supports the resilience needed to face the often stressful and demanding work of a PA. In contrast, when healthcare professionals do not care for their own holistic wellness, they are at increased risk for professional burnout.

Professional burnout is an emotional response to the long-term stress of work. In order to maintain a balanced life and good physical and mental health, and avoid professional burnout, PAs must show a commitment to themselves.

In an early version of CanMEDS, the role of the person was considered for inclusion as one of the domains in the framework; it was ultimately discarded as a role on its own.[14] One of the purposes of the person role was to encourage physicians to lead a holistically balanced and healthy life; to take care of themselves. The person role was also intended to acknowledge the physician's individuality and selfness in professional practice. Some of the elements of the person role, those related to self-care, were later folded into the professional role. Folding the person role into the professional role raises the question of whether sufficient value is placed on the personhood and well-being of the physician or PA. Interestingly, it was medical students who originally recognized the importance of the individuality and self-care of physicians, during the early development of CanMEDS.[14]

A few educational institutions recognized the prominent value of self-care and made a deliberate decision to include the person role or a similar domain. In the Netherlands, the role of reflection/reflector has been incorporated into medical training.[14] In the Ottawa University undergraduate medical program ePortfolio, the role of person as retained.[15]

Burnout

The widely applied Maslach Burnout Inventory tool[16] describes three dimensions of burnout: emotional exhaustion, depersonalization (also described as a cynical outlook), and a reduced sense of personal accomplishment or efficacy. Physical and emotional symptoms, such as physical exhaustion, headaches, sleeplessness, anxiety, depression, and anger, can also be associated with burnout.[17,18]

As of 2014, more than half of physicians in the United States experienced symptoms of burnout.[19] In Canada, a recent study by the Canadian Medical Association reported high levels of burnout in physicians.[20] In its startling findings, about a third of Canadian physicians reported feeling burned out or depressed, and 8% thought about suicide in the past year. The worst affected were medical residents, physicians in their first years of practice, and female physicians. The literature suggests that physician and nursing burnout is increasing.[19,21]

From the perspective of health professionals, burnout is associated with decreased satisfaction with work, a poor work-life balance, increased substance abuse, and increase physical and emotional illness, including suicidal ideation. For patients and the community, health professional burnout is associated with adverse results, such as increased medical errors and staff turnover.

A recent landmark meta-analysis showed convincingly that burnout is associated with increased negative patient outcomes, including unsafe care, unprofessional behavior, and low patient satisfaction of care. The greatest impact on these patient outcomes was related to the depersonalization feature of burnout.[22] Although this meta-analysis specifically focused on physicians, burnout can be found among PAs and other healthcare professionals.[17,23–25] This research draws a straight line between the well-being of healthcare professionals, and patient safety and quality of care. This finding should sound alarm bells for policy makers and all stakeholders (ie, everyone).

The situation for PAs is a little better.[26] PAs in the United States are less affected by symptoms of burnout compared with physicians, and they tend to have a more optimistic view of their work-life balance. However, exhaustion and stress from work are a serious concern, and these tend to peak in PAs with five to nine years of work experience. Interestingly, this same group of PAs report the highest rates of professional fulfillment, at 72.8%.

Avoiding or managing burnout is not an easy process. However, steps can, and should, be taken to prevent it from happening in the first place and addressing it promptly if it does occur. On an individual level, this can be done by combining habits of self-care, reflective practice, and active continued focus on resilience. On an institutional and systems level, careful thought and resources must be invested in ensuring that healthcare workers have the support needed.

THE TROUBLE WITH PROFESSIONALISM

Although CanMEDS-PA, the American Competencies for PAs, and other frameworks offer possible approaches to defining and describing professionalism, as previously discussed, the term is still notoriously difficult to pin down. At times, health professionals try to define it by its absence; they believe they know what it is when they do not see it. At other times, as in these competency frameworks, they include a list of adjectives to describe characteristics that, taken together, seem to add up to professional behavior. They use language like honesty, integrity, commitment, compassion, altruism, accountability, ethical decision making, respect for diversity, privacy and confidentiality, adherence to the laws and regulations of practice, appropriate grooming and attire, and so on. On their surface, these all seem fitting and desirable professional traits; characteristics becoming of a PA. Many of these attitudinal attributes were included in the definitions discussed earlier. However, in developing their working definition, Cruess and colleagues[4] argue that "a list of attributes, characteristics, or behavioral patterns is too broad to serve as [a definition]."[4(p75)]

Although it is valuable, on one level, to identify professional behavior with these traits and characteristics, there are a few challenges to limiting the definition of professionalism with this approach, which are considered here. First, in the context of competency-based education and practice, these characteristics do not lend themselves readily to observation, teaching, learning, and assessment. Even if PAs try to identify and assess them, they cannot be sure whether the display of professionalism is authentic and sustainable or simply a superficial display for social acceptance or to please faculty and receive a favorable professionalism assessment grade.[27]

Second, and closely related to the first challenge, is that evaluating professional behavior is highly subjective and context dependent, making its identification and assessment even more difficult. Third, some of the characteristics used to describe professional behavior may seem obvious and acceptable on their surface but are more complex and fraught on further reflection. One such characteristic that is usually accepted at face value as a positive professional characteristic is altruism. Even this seemingly respectable professional trait is more complex and fraught on deeper inspection. In addition, professionalism goes beyond describing individual healthcare providers and their personal traits; it extends to the character and position of the entire profession within society.

In the current professional landscape, observable behaviors are the key to defining and assessing competence during training and through a PA's career. PA educators agree that professional behavior cannot be assessed easily, based on, for example, a written test or itemized checklist. Professionalism is one of the areas of competence that challenges healthcare educators to develop appropriate curricular content and assessment tools. In one study, investigators showed that there is little agreement even among clinical educators regarding the appropriate response to professionally challenging situations.[28] In some clinical case scenarios, faculty had different, sometimes conflicting, responses regarding how medical trainees should respond to a professionally challenging situation. If practicing clinical faculty are not able to agree on what professional behavior is, how can professionalism even be taught or assessed? This study also showed that, although clinical faculty often agreed on the underlying values in a case scenario (eg, the need to balance patient autonomy with patient safety), their methods of expressing these values varied significantly (eg, telling the truth at all costs vs temporarily withholding some information to protect a patient's well-being). This finding is illuminating and instructive, because it highlights the situational, context-specific nature of professional behavior. After all, the goal is to train PAs who are guided by underlying values, with the wisdom to act in ways that reflect those values, rather than training PAs who will indiscriminately behave in the same way, with little regard to situation and context.

To round out the discussion of defining and applying the traits and values underpinning professionalism, it is helpful to consider David Stern's[29] definition, in which he emphasizes the observable aspects of professionalism, which is the best that can be achieved in teaching, learning, and assessing professionalism. He says, "Professionalism is demonstrated through a foundation of clinical competence, communication skills, and ethical understanding, upon which is built the aspiration to and wise application of the principles of professionalism: excellence, humanism, accountability, and altruism."[29] These four principles of professionalism (excellence, humanism, accountability, and altruism) offer a framework that may be specific and concrete enough to be of practical use in practice and in education.

A few specific characteristics and attitudes related to professionalism, and new insights related to these traits, are discussed next.

ALTRUISM

Altruism is a professional characteristic that may not be as straightforward as it first appears. Altruism has long been associated, almost synonymous, with the healthcare professions. As mentioned earlier, the American competency profile for PAs[30] defines professionalism as "the expression of positive values and ideals as care is delivered" and adds that, "Foremost, it involves prioritizing the interests of those being served above one's own." It is true that caring for others is at the core of healthcare; after all, it is called health *care*. However, some have argued that altruism may go too far; that altruism, with its specific usage in medicine, has been socially constructed to imply self-sacrifice; putting the needs of the patient before clinicians' own needs and self-interest, sometimes to the detriment of the self. The literature of the so-called hidden curriculum in medical education often highlights this point. Although this is not taught in the formal medical school curriculum, the hidden curriculum sometimes rewards physicians who neglect self-care activities, such as sleep, nutrition, and leisure activity. The effects of excessive altruism are burnout and detachment, caused by self-sacrifice, overwork, and stress.[31] These reactions have further negative effects on the well-being of the medical learners, as well as on their empathy and professionalism, and even on patient safety.[22,32,33] Going beyond the call of duty was once the expected norm in medicine, rather than the exception. At least, this was true for the baby-boomer generation; attitudes seem to be shifting in generation X, who seem to have a lower regard for the concept of altruism in medical practice.[34]

This constructed usage of altruism as self-sacrifice, although widely accepted and even once promoted, has a paradoxic effect. Excessive altruism directly opposes another imperative of professional behavior that has, rightly, received increasing attention in recent decades; that of self-care. How can these seemingly opposing values be reconciled? How can clinicians put the needs of patients ahead of their own needs, and at the same time care for their own health and well-being?

Bishop and Rees[34] propose the term prosocial behavior instead of altruism as a more specific description of the desirable professional trait. Using prosocial behavior simultaneously promotes both beneficence to the patient and self-care, addressing the inherent conflict of altruism, described earlier. Furthermore, it lends itself more readily to observable behavior, and therefore to teaching and assessment. Prosocial behavior resonates well with the CanMEDS-PA definition of professionalism presented earlier, which includes "the promotion of public good."[1(p21)]

One practical way to consider the balance between the needs of patients and the needs of PAs is to reflect on the distinction between a PA's personal preference and what is needed to preserve the PA's own health and well-being. Self-care is in the category of needs. It seems appropriate that practicing PAs would consider prioritizing a patient's needs over their own personal preferences, but the PAs would also be right to prioritize their own well-being. The challenge is the "gray zone" where the line between a need and a preference is not clear, or when the needs of the patient and the PA are at odds.

For example, consider a scenario in which a patient, Saira, arrives late for a clinic appointment, just as the office is about to close for the day. The PA, Jim, has an important family event to attend. It is his grandmother's 80th birthday dinner party. The entire extended family will be there, even guests who flew in from across the country. Everyone is looking forward to seeing Jim; the expectation is that he will be there, and on time. The PA tells Saira that he cannot stay late. Just then, Saira becomes very emotional and begins to cry. She communicates that she is distraught because of a family crisis. Should Jim ask Saira to reschedule an appointment, or should he stay late to talk with Saira and miss a portion of the family party, knowing how disappointed they will be when he arrives late, as usual? Based on the author's own past teaching experience, I guess that about half the readers think Jim should stay, and half think he should leave and ask Saira to come back another day.

There is no right or wrong answer to this question; it is meant as a thought exercise. It depends on the context and, of course, the details. For one thing, in what state is the patient? Is Saira depressed and potentially at risk of self-harm? Is there an immediate crisis or is this a recurring issue? Jim needs to weigh the acuity of the patient's need with his own needs. What are his own attitudes toward self-care? Would missing this event cost him, in terms of his personal relationships or his own protected leisure time? Is he already feeling burned out from staying many late nights after hours? Is there a patient safety issue, which should never be ignored? Is there a risk to Jim's well-being?

To show the importance of self-care, consider the analogy to the coronary circulation. The heart is responsible for delivering oxygenated blood to all the organs and tissues. It must pump with enough force and volume to reach the narrowest capillaries in the most distal regions, but the heart cannot function effectively without supplying its own coronary circulation. If there is an interruption in the blood flow of the heart's circulation by a clot or by narrowing of the vessels, this can damage the heart, and the heart may not be able to do its job of effectively circulating blood to the rest of the body. If the heart cannot take care of itself, it will not be able to care for the rest of the body. Similarly, if PAs do not care for themselves, they will not be able to effectively provide care for their patients. The heart must serve both itself and the body. PAs must care for themselves and for their patients. It is not one or the other; it is both. The paradox is resolved with a focus on self-care in the context of service, as discussed next.

SERVICE

Service is an attitude in healthcare that has not received much attention lately, and that perhaps deserves a revival. Many medical learners arrive on the scene with a service-oriented attitude, which diminishes during their education.[32] The term service seems to have gone out of style in society; in healthcare, in politics, and beyond. The emphasis on personal autonomy and self-determination seems to render modern Western society averse to connotations of subservience. The ideas of service may be even more distasteful to PAs because of their specific scope of practice, which limits their independent decision making and may imply deference to their supervising physicians.

Autonomy and self-determination have positive social benefits. They are foundational values in a democratic society and support aspiration-based and merit-based social advancement. However, a service-oriented attitude also has its merits. In arguing that experts, such as medical professionals, are struggling to maintain their authority in society, Tom Nichols[35] concludes by saying that "experts need to remember, always, that they are the servants and not the master of a democratic society…"[35] Regarding their clinical practice as a form of service to their patients only adds meaning to their work. This orientation helps them better understand their role within their delivery of care, neither overvaluing nor undervaluing their position. It is a way to describe their relative position to their patients and to the public, and to proudly honor that position.

This approach does not minimize the caring aspect of healthcare, nor does it suggest that PAs' work is composed of mere technical or delegated tasks. On the contrary, it is to reimagine what PAs do, in a way that honors both the patients and the providers, much in the way the term prosocial behavior does.[34] Providing care in service to patients implies acknowledging the patients' role as the beneficiary of clinicians' compassion and expertise, and, at the same time, acknowledging the value of the care that is provided and the expertise that is offered, care that can only be provided by PAs when they care for themselves and are well and whole.

This situation can be compared with politicians who acknowledges their role as public servants. This framing serves to elevate both the public and the role of the politicians and give them mutual context. Medicine and politics both aspire to the altruistic ideals of service, beneficence, giving, and sacrifice, but both have potential pitfalls and the risk of succumbing to ulterior motives, such as financial gain, respect, status, and power. Although altruism cannot be observed or measured, service lends itself more readily to observable outcomes. No one can ever know what motivates someone to act; even in a situation that seems entirely altruistic, there may be selfish motivations, such as fame or honor. However, acting in service to patients shows self-respect, and respect for the patients and society. It honors both the role of the patients and that of the PAs. Rather than diminishing either, it elevates both.

COMPASSION

Compassion, care, sympathy, empathy, altruism. Why so many words? Humans are driven toward prosocial attitudes and behaviors. There are many different ways to consider these similar and overlapping elements. There is considerable evidence that humans have evolved to nurture and protect each other, especially their young, in order to support themselves as a species. However, there exist competing selfish motivations and behaviors. Clearly, not everyone shows prosocial attitudes and behaviors; very few do so consistently and without exception. (Just imagine yourself, normally compassionate and caring, behind the wheel in heavy traffic, maybe late for a shift, being cut off by an aggressive driver in the next lane.)

PAs are motivated, in large part, by their willingness to provide care and compassion to their patients. This gives their lives meaning and satisfaction. Were they born with these attitudes and motivations? Did they learn them somewhere, in childhood or in PA school? Are they somehow inadvertently unlearning them along the way? To understand the answers to these questions, it is helpful to understand how these attitudes and behaviors are seen through various lenses.

The word compassion is derived from Latin and means to suffer with, or together. What is immediately striking in this definition is that expressing compassion does not necessarily involve an action. Compassion can, and should, move or motivate PAs to take action to alleviate a patient's suffering or need; however, compassion in itself is simply sharing in the pain or need of another. They can do something, even without doing anything. Sometimes, when they are at a loss and unable to alleviate a patient's suffering or pain, because they do not know what is causing it, or because there is no effective treatment, they can contemplate the simple meaning of the word compassion and understand that there is something they can do to help: just be with the patient and share in the patient's pain or suffering.

One definition of compassion is "the feeling that arises in witnessing another's suffering and that motivates a subsequent desire to help."[36(p2)] This definition focuses on compassion as a complex, but discrete, emotional response.[37(p3)] The concern for the other is coupled with the desire to alleviate the suffering or provide the unmet need. This definition distinguishes compassion from empathy; the latter being a broader term that refers to the general ability to appreciate or share the feelings of another.

Other conceptions of compassion describe it not as an emotional state, but as a core motivation, a personality trait or disposition, or as an attitude. From the perspective of compassion as a core motivation, compassion is seen as a basic human drive to provide care. This view seems to emphasize the drive to provide care from the subjective feelings of sharing emotionally in the suffering of others. As a personality trait, compassion can be viewed in terms of its consistency and stability over time: how likely someone is to show compassion.

Does it matter how compassion is defined; as an emotional state, a stable personality trait, a core motivation, or an attitude? It matters, because thinking of these different ways of conceptualizing compassion can help PAs understand how to enhance and develop this element in the care they provide. As an emotion, PAs can reflect on times they experienced these feelings and consider how they act and react. As a personality trait, PA Programs can consider the implications on the PA education admissions process. Should programs target applicants who show this trait? Or can they readily teach their otherwise brilliant students how to show compassion? Should PAs who are highly compassionate use this insight to guide their chosen field of practice? Would they do especially well in an area of care that is compassion heavy, such as palliative care or oncology? Or would this lead them to early burnout because of their tendency to feel the pain of others?

CARING

It would seem that care is a predominant component of every health profession. However, the terms care and caring are notoriously ambiguous and resistant to simple definitions. Perhaps more than any other concept in healthcare, care and caring can also be understood differently from different professional perspectives. Among the health professions, nursing is most closely linked with the term caring. In nursing, caring (with a lower case c) can be distinguished by the type of activities done by friends and loved ones, to show concern and support, versus Caring (with an upper case C) as the professional activities provided by nurses. The former is characterized by kindness, concern, neighborliness, looking after, and doing for, in the context of the types of activities friends, family, and loved ones do for one another. The latter is characterized by professional activity provided by nurses in the context of their clinical skills and theoretic knowledge base (Jocelyn Bennet, Director, AMS Phoenix Project, email communication, 2019).

There are several barriers to compassionate care, including time pressures, fatigue, burnout, and organizational limitations.

Several multidisciplinary projects and symposia have been organized in recent years to address the perceived lack of care and humanism in healthcare delivery in several North American and European countries. A few such organizations devoted to this effort are the AMS Phoenix Project in Canada, the Arnold P. Gold Foundation in the United States, and the Leadership in Compassionate Care Program in the United Kingdom. These initiatives point to the dual reality that there is a need to improve the care and humanism across the health professions and that there is a deep interest and motivation in achieving this goal.

Can Care and Compassion Be Taught?

Question that emerges regularly in admissions committees for health professions educational programs are: what are the essential qualities to be identified in applicants and what are the qualities that can be taught during the course of study? If kindness and compassion are considered traits that can be taught and learned, then why is it necessary to select these qualities in incoming students? In contrast, if these are innate characteristics that are resistant to change, such as personality types, what is the purpose of teaching attitudes of kindness and compassion? People either have it or they do not. The answer probably lies somewhere in the middle. If, indeed, kind, compassionate, humanistic PAs are wanted, these characteristics should first be identified and selected in the admissions process and, second, these attitudes should be re-enforced and promoted longitudinally through the educational program. If these characteristics are to be promoted as foundational to the PA profession, the profession should accept caring, compassionate students and strengthen and promote these values throughout their education. However, it has been documented that medical students may actually decline over the course of their preclinical and clinical training in their attitudes toward relational aspects of practice. These declining attitudes include appreciation of patients' social determinants of health, attitudes toward preventive health and interprofessional collaboration, and recognizing the importance of the doctor-patient relationship.[38]

The relevant question may not be whether care and compassion can be taught, but how best to re-enforce, promote and support these attributes in educational programs and in clinical practice settings. Furthermore, how can barriers that prevent care and compassion be removed, and how can the profession ensure that these values and attitudes are not unlearned in these carefully selected students?

How, then, can humanistic characteristics be supported and promoted during the education process? A few suggestions that have been proposed include lifelong learning and refresher courses for clinicians in practice, positive role modeling, early clinical exposure, and simulation learning with feedback.[37(pp468,469)]

CONSCIENTIOUSNESS

Conscientiousness is one of the so-called big five personality traits[39]; traits that are considered stable through a person's lifetime. Conscientiousness predicts several measures of success and well-being, such as academic performance,[40] lower lifetime unemployment,[41] and the ability to recover from negative emotions.[42] Conscientiousness reflects dependability, carefulness, thoroughness, responsibility, and organization. Some scholars have also suggested that this trait includes being hard working, achievement oriented, and persevering.[43] In the NEO Personality Inventory-3, the facets of conscientiousness include competence, order, dutifulness, achievement striving, self-discipline, and deliberation.[39]

Based on this description, it is no wonder that conscientious personality traits are desirable in PAs and any other healthcare provider. Most people would want their own care providers to reflect these qualities.

In 2012, the University of Toronto Council of Health Sciences Education Subcommittee held a retreat, Innovations and Boundless Directions: Health Professions Education Reforms, which brought together faculty across the health science education programs. The objective of this retreat was to advance the priorities of the 2010 report, "Health Professionals for a New Century: Transforming Education to Strengthen Health Systems in an Interdependent World."[44] One key direction of the retreat was to pilot initiatives to identify common noncognitive characteristics desirable in candidates for all health professions, and to potentially develop some collaborative admissions processes. The rationale was based on the supposition that all healthcare professions' education programs are looking for specific characteristics in their applicants, and that some of these characteristics are likely common across the professions. A modified Delphi technique was used to collect and prioritize the characteristics suggested by an interprofessional group of faculty members from across the health science programs. The group recommendation was to explore the attributes of conscientiousness, communicativeness, and ethical practice, in that order. Interestingly, conscientiousness was the number one characteristic that was at the top of the list among this interprofessional group of faculty members. An ideal PA is both caring and conscientious. Each of these characteristics, on its own, is important. Together, they are a "dream team" of professional attributes.

SUMMARY

Professionalism is a highly valued concept in the PA profession and in all health professions. There are many definitions and descriptions of what it means to be a professional. This multitude of definitions is an indication of the complex nature of professionalism. Some of the more useful descriptions identify professionalism as a set of values that reflect the profession, as well as a set of individual traits and characteristics that individual PAs should embody.

Professionalism is shown through the commitment of PAs in four domains: commitment to the patient, the profession, the public, and to self. Commitment to the patient implies excellence in the knowledge, skills, and attitudes of PAs, as expressed in every patient encounter. Commitment to the profession implies identification with, and involvement in, professional organizations and professional advocacy. Commitment to the public is achieved through honoring the PA profession's social contract: adhering to the responsibilities of the profession, living up to the public's trust, and enjoying the privileges of this status. Commitment to self involves prioritizing self-care and valuing holistic health of mind, body, and spirit. PAs must care for their own well-being in order to effectively provide care throughout a long career and avoid professional burnout.

Several specific characteristics are also associated with professionalism, including altruism, service, compassion, caring, and conscientiousness. This article explores these characteristics to gain insight into their relationship to each other and to the professional landscape. Gaining a deeper understanding into this challenging aspect of PA practice can have a significant impact on how PAs practice as healthcare professionals.

ACKNOWLEDGMENTS

The author would like to thank the Consortium of PA Education, the Department of Family & Community Medicine, and the University of Toronto for supporting the preparation of this article.

REFERENCES

1. CanMEDS-PA. 2015. Ottawa (Canada): Canadian Association of Physician Assistants. Available at: https://capa-acam.ca/wp-content/uploads/2015/11/CanMEDS-PA.pdf.
2. Competencies for the Physician Assistant Profession. https://www.aapa.org/wp-content/uploads/2017/02/PA-Competencies-updated.pdf.
3. Profession, n. Oxford University Press.
4. Cruess SR, Johnston S, Cruess RL. "Profession": a working definition for medical educators. Teach Learn Med 2004;16(1):74–6.

5. CAPA Code of Ethics. Canadian Association of Physician Assistants. 2016. Available at: https://capa-acam.ca/wp-content/uploads/2016/02/Code-of-Ethics_Feb_2016_FINAL.pdf. Accessed January 15, 2019.

6. Martimianakis MA, Maniate JM, Hodges BD. Sociological interpretations of professionalism. Med Educ 2009;43(9):829–37.

7. Friedson E. Professional dominance: the social structure of medical care. New York: Atherton Press; 1970.

8. Starr P. The social transformation of American medicine. 6th edition 2017.

9. Cruess SR. Professionalism and medicine's social contract with society. Clin Orthop Relat Res 2006;449:170–6.

10. Buchman S, Woollard R, Meili R, et al. Practising social accountability. Can Fam Physician 2016;62(1):15.

11. Goel R, Buchman S, Meili R, et al. Social accountability at the micro level. Can Fam Physician 2016;62(4):287.

12. Meili R, Buchman S, Goel R, et al. Social accountability at the macro level. Can Fam Physician 2016;62(10):785.

13. Woollard R, Buchman S, Meili R, et al. Social accountability at the meso level. Can Fam Physician 2016;62(7):538.

14. Whitehead C, Selleger V, Kreeke J, et al. The 'missing person' in roles-based competency models: a historical, cross-national, contrastive case study. Med Educ 2014;48(8):785–95.

15. University of Ottawa Faculty of Medicine ePortfolio. Available at: https://www.med.uottawa.ca/ePortfolio/.

16. Maslach C, Jackson SE. The measurement of experienced burnout. J Organ Behav 1981;2(2):99–113.

17. Cañadas-De la Fuente GA, Vargas C, San Luis C, et al. Risk factors and prevalence of burnout syndrome in the nursing profession. Int J Nurs Stud 2015;52(1): 240–9.

18. Shanafelt TD, Boone S, Tan L, et al. Burnout and satisfaction with work-life balance among US physicians relative to the general US population burnout and satisfaction with work-life balance. JAMA Intern Med 2012;172(18):1377–85.

19. Shanafelt TD, Hasan O, Dyrbye LN, et al. Changes in burnout and satisfaction with work-life balance in physicians and the general US working population between 2011 and 2014. Mayo Clin Proc 2015;90(12):1600–13.

20. CMA national physician health survey: a national snapshot. 2018. Available at: https://www.cma.ca/Assets/assets-library/document/en/advocacy/nph-survey-e.pdf. Accessed November 18, 2018.

21. Employee engagement in nursing survey. Kronos Incorporated; 2017. Available at: https://www.kronos.com/about-us/newsroom/kronos-survey-finds-nurses-love-what-they-do-though-fatigue-pervasive-problem.

22. Panagioti M, Geraghty K, Johnson J, et al. Association between physician burnout and patient safety, professionalism, and patient satisfaction: a systematic review and meta-analysis. JAMA Intern Med 2018;178(10):1317–30.

23. Altun I. Burnout and nurses' personal and professional values. Nurs Ethics 2002; 9(3):269–78.

24. Benson MAP, Peterson TE, Salazar LMS, et al. Burnout in rural physician assistants: an initial study. J Physician Assist Educ 2016;27(2):81–3.

25. Tetzlaff ED, Hylton HM, DeMora L, et al. National study of burnout and career satisfaction among physician assistants in oncology: implications for team-based care. J Oncol Pract 2018;14(1):e11–22.

26. Smith N. Are PAs burned out?. 2018. Available at: https://www.aapa.org/news-central/2018/05/pas-report-low-burnout/. Accessed November 18, 2018.
27. Hafferty FW. Measuring professionalism: a commentary. New York: Oxford University Press; 2006.
28. Ginsburg S, Regehr G, Lingard L. Basing the evaluation of professionalism on observable behaviors: a cautionary tale. Research in Medical Education Proceedings of the Forty-Third Annual Conference November 7-10. Acad Med 2004;79(10):S1–4.
29. Stern DT. Measuring medical professionalism. New York: Oxford University Press; 2006.
30. Competencies for the physician assistant profession. JAAPA 2005;18(7):16–8. Available at: http://link.galegroup.com.myaccess.library.utoronto.ca/apps/doc/A160711804/AONE?u=utoronto_main&sid=AONE&xid=279e0ace.
31. Dyrbye LN, Shanafelt TD. Commentary: medical student distress: a call to action. Acad Med 2011;86(7):801–3.
32. Hafferty FW. What medical students know about professionalism. Mt Sinai J Med 2002;69(6):385–97.
33. Thomas MR, Dyrbye LN, Huntington JL, et al. How do distress and well-being relate to medical student empathy? A multicenter study. J Gen Intern Med 2007;22(2):177–83.
34. Bishop JP, Rees CE. Hero or has-been: Is there a future for altruism in medical education? Adv Health Sci Educ Theor Pract 2007;12(3):391–9.
35. Nichols TM. The death of expertise: the campaign against established knowledge and why it matters. New York: Oxford University Press, Inc; 2017.
36. Goetz JL, Keltner D, Simon-Thomas E. Compassion: an evolutionary analysis and empirical review. Psychol Bull 2010;136(3):351–74.
37. Seppala E, Simon-Thomas E, Brown SL, et al. The Oxford handbook of compassion science. New York: Oxford University Press; 2017.
38. Woloschuk W, Harasym PH, Temple W. Attitude change during medical school: a cohort study. Med Educ 2004;38(5):522–34.
39. Costa PT, McCrae RR. Normal personality assessment in clinical practice: the NEO personality inventory. Psychol Assess 1992;4(1):5–13.
40. Vianello M, Robusto E, Anselmi P. Implicit conscientiousness predicts academic performance. Personal Individual Differences 2010;48(4):452–7.
41. Egan M, Daly M, Delaney L, et al. Adolescent conscientiousness predicts lower lifetime unemployment. J Appl Psychol 2017;102(4):700–9.
42. Javaras KN, Schaefer SM, van Reekum CM, et al. Conscientiousness predicts greater recovery from negative emotion. Emotion 2012;12(5):875–81.
43. Barrick MR, Mount MK. The big five personality dimensions and job performance: a meta-analysis. Personnel Psychology 1991;44(1):1–26.
44. Frenk J, Chen L, Bhutta ZA, et al. Health professionals for a new century: transforming education to strengthen health systems in an interdependent world. Lancet 2010;376(9756):1923–58.

Reflective Practice for Physician Assistants

Sharona Kanofsky, PA-C, CCPA, MScCH

KEYWORDS

• Healthcare • Medicine • Physician Assistant • Reflection • Reflective practice

KEY POINTS

- Reflection is a higher-order metacognitive process that allows a Physician Assistant (PA) to identify and analyze individual challenges in practice, with the purpose of addressing these challenges.
- The process of reflection allows the PA to develop actionable plans to address the gaps in current knowledge, skills, or attitudes.
- Reflection is derived from the education psychology theories of reflective practice but has shifted from its theoretic foundations to its common use in healthcare education and practice.

INTRODUCTION

You may have come across a bumper sticker or coffee mug emblazoned with these words erroneously attributed to Mahatma Gandhi: "Be the change that you wish to see in the world."[1] Healthcare providers start with a desire to change the world for the better. We may feel conflicted, even discouraged, when we discover that the scope of our influence is less than we hoped. Our lofty make-the-world-a-better-place aspirations are stymied by seemingly opposing forces and mundane obstacles: local and governmental rules and regulations; our patients' own socioeconomic context or degree of motivation; complex clinical problems that defy easy solutions; our own physical, mental, and emotional limits; and many more.

This quote about "being the change" reminds us that there *is* always something we can do to make the world a better place. We can make a dedicated effort to think about, to *reflect* upon, the healthcare system in which we work and our own clinical practice. Sometimes this requires a critical view or out-of-the-box thinking: questioning norms and assumptions about the healthcare system and about ourselves or reimagining ways of approaching challenges. We can, and should, make concerted, organized, and regular efforts to think about and improve these systems and our own practices through reflection.

Faculty of Medicine, Department of Family and Community Medicine, Physician Assistant Program, 263 McCaul Street, 3rd Floor, Toronto, Ontario, M5T 1W7, Canada
E-mail address: sharona.kanofsky@utoronto.ca

Physician Assist Clin 5 (2020) 27–37
https://doi.org/10.1016/j.cpha.2019.08.003
2405-7991/20/© 2019 Elsevier Inc. All rights reserved.

Reflection is a component of both the American and Canadian PA competency profiles. The American competencies list self-reflection in the Professionalism domain,[2] (p. 17) whereas the Canadian competency profile, CanMEDS-PA, lists reflection in the Scholar role. An argument can clearly be made for both. Reflection is a feature of a PA's professionalism, as a trait related to self-awareness and even self-care. Reflection is also a feature of a PA as a scholar, in the sense that this habit of mind is used to determine areas for learning and continuing professional development.

WHAT IS REFLECTION?

What is reflection? Reflection is often referred to as a *metacognitive process*—it involves thinking about thinking. But as we shall see, it goes beyond simply thinking about how we think, although this is an important feature. Reflection also involves thinking about how we behave and perform in practice. One definition of reflection describes it as "a metacognitive process that occurs before, during, and after situations with the purpose of developing greater understanding of both the self and the situation so that future encounters with the situation are informed from previous encounters."[3] (p. 685) This definition implies that the reflective process, although itself a cognitive exercise, is intended for the practical purpose of informing and improving future performance.

Habits of reflection should be developed early in PA education, as these habits represent foundational attitudes and skills of a competent PA. The goal is to ingrain these habits and refine the related skill set through day to day practice, so that it becomes second-nature, regular, and routine.

Joseph Kennedy, the father of US President John F. Kennedy, famously criticized his son's political opponent in 1960, during the presidential race: "I continually hear about Nixon's experience and I certainly think, for the most part, that experience is a term used to describe a lifetime of mistakes."[4] Or put another way, "Ten years of experience without reflection is just one year experience repeated ten times."[5] (p. 139) It is true that we can do the same thing, over and over, for many years, and imagine that we are getting better at it by gaining experience. However, if we are making errors or otherwise missing the intended mark, and we lack a reliable process by which to identify and address these gaps, we may only be reinforcing and ingraining these errors in practice. We are repeatedly missing opportunities to build on our areas of competency. We may not be getting better at competent PA practice; we may only be getting better at our mistakes.

For a practicing PA, especially, there is probably no greater an asset than the ability to know your own abilities and limitations. Reflection relies on the open attitude of acknowledging individual challenges and barriers and having the will to address them. Your collaborating physicians and other healthcare team members will be able to trust that you know what you can competently manage and recognize when you need to reach out for support from a physician or other team members. This type of insight underpins the physician-PA relationship.

THEORETIC BACKGROUND OF REFLECTION: REFLECTION AND REFLECTIVE PRACTICE

Reflective practice, as an area of study, is derived from the philosophy of education and came about as an alternative, or complement, to what were at the time the dominant forms of knowledge—scientific knowledge, evidence-based practice, and technical rationality. Reflection developed as an alternate form of knowledge to these previously dominant forms—an epistemology of practice—that acknowledged the uncertainty, uniqueness, and value conflicts in Schön's "intermediate zones of prac-tice," as described later.[6] (p. 6). Reflective practice allows us to be "resilient in the face of adversity and receptive in the face of uncertainty."[7]

The two main strands of theories of Reflection and Reflective Practice that emerged from the earlier work describe (1) an epistemology of practice and (2) a critical social theory. The first strand, epistemology of practice, describes what practitioners actu-ally do when they work. It reflects the artistic and iterative processes of a professional at work, such as the application of tacit knowledge, improvisation, and reflection-in-action. The second strand, critical social theory, uses a deconstructive lens of critical social inquiry to shine light on areas of social structure and question the status quo, using professionals as agents of social change.

Medical education literature often conflates the terms *reflection* and *reflective practice*. Although they are closely related, the author distinguishes between them, in an effort to use language accurately and to situate reflective practice in its theoretic foundations. Stella Ng distinguished these two concepts as follows: "Reflection is a way of thinking, which may manifest itself in learning, practice, or in one's way of being. Reflective practice is a way of theorizing about the embodied and tacit, and intentional and explicit, forms of reflection within professional practice."[8]

In healthcare and in healthcare education, reflection and reflective practice have mostly become synonymous. The common use of the term *reflective practice* has moved away from its theoretic roots and toward the application of the metacognitive process of reflection that helps us make sense of things that occur in practice and consider ways to improve the quality of care. Reflection in healthcare education and practice has also, erroneously, become conflated with self-reflection. Although thinking critically about one's own practice and ways to improve our own performance is a valuable pursuit, it should be noted that this focus on the self is not at the core of the original theories of reflective practice.[7]

THE ART OF MEDICINE

You may have heard the expression that medicine is not just a science; it is an art. Referring to the practice of medicine as an art may seem strange at first. Clearly, it is not what we typically think of as either fine or performing art, such as painting, sculp-ture, drama, or dance. You may have a vague sense of what this idea implies or the message it attempts to convey, but let us examine this expression more closely to get a fuller perspective. How exactly is medicine a form of art?

In fact, what could be more rooted in science than the practice of medicine? The modern tradition of medicine rests on a deep and detailed understanding of how the human body works—the mechanics of joint movements; the pharmacologic effects of medications on tissues and organs; the multitude of biochemical reac-tions at the cellular level; the electrical circuitry of the heart, and so on. Medicine is a deeply scientific pursuit. There exist many guidelines, for treatment, diagnosis, screening, and prevention, which are based on scientific research and reproduc-ible, predictable results in defined populations and clinical scenarios. For a moment, one might imagine that medicine is really a series of technical challenges with instrumental solutions, guided by medical research and sound scientific pro-cesses. Whatever the medical question, science will have an answer that we can use to fix our patients' problems.

But of course, we know this is not at all the way medicine works. The technical and scientific knowledge and skills learned in PA school, or any health profession educational program, at times seem insufficient to address complex, real-world problems. Donald Schön, one of the early thinkers on reflective practice, described the topography of professional practice as "a high, hard ground overlooking a swamp."[6] [(p. 3)] He describes how research-based techniques may be adequate to address simpler "high ground" issues that arise in practice. However, when issues become more complex, they resemble more of a swampy terrain and the simple solutions no longer apply. The dilemma he presents, then, is: how can practitioners, such as PAs, be adequately educated and prepared for the real world of complex, "swampy" problems, if these complex problems only present themselves in real world settings?

One way this is addressed in many practice fields is by placing students in the real world of practice, as in PA training, with clinical placements as the focus of the second year in most programs. But even the clinical placement is not a place where the PA is actually *doing* the work of a PA, but rather learning *how* to do the work of a PA. Schön refers to the abovementioned real-world complexities as "intermediate zones of practice" that are identifiable through their defining features—uncertainty, uniqueness, and value conflict.[6] [(p. 6)] One cannot simply apply the instrumental tools of theory and scientific knowledge learned in the classroom to these types of complex clinical problems. Paradoxically, one can really only learn to solve these complex problems *while* solving them.

This type of higher-order learning through practice can be achieved through reflective practice, and this explains why medicine can be described as an art. *The only way to learn to do art is by doing it.* In other words, beyond theory and technical knowledge, the creative act is one of trial and correction. What an artist may try, and retry, is based on his own judgment of his work. A form or an image may emerge from the medium that does not quite match the intended image in the artist's mind's eye. Then the artist will revisit the technique, the stroke of the wrist, the choice of color or texture, and try again with some slight adjustment to get it right, or closer to what was intended, with each iteration. Similarly, in the practice of medicine, there are almost always adjustments that can be made to improve a PA's performance, and these can also be done through the process of reflection.

An experienced artist cannot always explain or deconstruct how she knew which adjustments would improve her sculpture; she just knew implicitly. She may not even be able to say *what* exact adjustments were made, how she changed the angle of her tool in her hand or how she adjusted the force of her carving. But she did it and did it well. This is called tacit or implicit knowledge and is sometimes described as "knowing how." It is the type of knowledge we attain without being able to explain exactly how we know it or even how to do it.

Tacit or implicit knowledge contrasts with explicit knowledge, which is the type of knowledge often learned from textbooks and lectures, information that can be easily identified and communicated. This type of knowledge can be described as "knowing that." Like the artist described earlier, an experienced PA also may not be able to explain the exact adjustments in voice modulation, eye contact, or body language made during a conversation with a patient. But these subtle adjustments allowed the patient to feel a greater sense of trust in that moment and perhaps share a personal and pertinent detail in the health history. The process of reflection-in-action guides the PA to do just that, in the moment. Reflection is a metacognitive activity that allows a PA to think about her thoughts and actions, analyze them, and make adjustments, sometimes even in the moment. Reflection aims to help the artist, or the PA, become more aware of her actions, by contemplating the tacit or implicit knowledge, and making it overt and explicit.

REFLECTION-IN-ACTION AND REFLECTION-ON-ACTION

Schön describes reflection at different stages of action: *Reflection-in-action* and *Reflection-on-action*. Earlier, the author gave examples of *reflection-in-action,* when the adjustments are made during the activity. This process can be both implicit and explicit. With the example of the artist or the PA in the previous section, the author described the process of adjustment being made subconsciously, based on deep experience and expertise.

Reflection-in-action can also occur explicitly, when the PA consciously considers what is happening while it is happening and makes adjustments accordingly. This process occurs regularly with competitive athletes, and this analogy can also be useful to consider. A competitive swimmer in a race is trained to assess her own performance while practicing and even while racing. She consciously considers her stroke mechanics, breathing, and exertion and makes adjustments in real time. A major league baseball player will review his swing in his mind after striking out and consider how to adjust his swing for the next at-bat, based on the types of pitches the pitcher is throwing. He will time up his pitches while on deck, as the batter ahead of him in the order takes his pitches. This is reflection-in-action. It may be conscious or subconscious and is usually a combination of both.

Reflection-in-action overlaps with the cognitive process of self-monitoring. Self-monitoring has been described as "slowing down when one should" and "knowing when to look it up."[9–10] It involves the ability to recognize a problem in the moment and realize the need to resolve it, either by slowing down to become more deliberate and careful or by seeking help when reaching the limit of one's abilities by looking up the information or asking a more expert clinician.

In contrast to reflection-in-action, which occurs during an activity or encounter, reflection-on-action occurs after the activity or encounter. This form of reflection relies on conscious consideration of an event or encounter. The PA will consider how an encounter played out, what happened, how, and why. The PA will attempt to create some meaningful lesson from the encounter and apply this lesson in similar encounters in the future. This is the type of reflection most commonly encountered in healthcare professional education and practice.

REFLECTION IN PHYSICIAN ASSISTANT EDUCATION

Reflection in healthcare education has largely veered away from the theoretic foundations of reflective practice and developed into a new form in teaching and assessment, with both positive and negative consequences. The overwhelming positive result of reflection in PA education is its focus on metacognition and the resulting emphasis on practice improvement and life-long learning. PA students often write enthusiastically in course feedback comments that learning about the reflective process has opened their eyes to a new way of thinking and made them more aware of the impact of what would otherwise seem to be mundane events. There is no doubt that these are good habits of mind that promote quality of care and personal and professional satisfaction.

On the other hand, there are pitfalls in this area of education. For example, using written reflective essays as course assessments risks undermining their authenticity and confusing the act of reflection with the act of writing about reflection. There may also be confusion over what is being considered in the reflection. What aspect is being assessed? Is it the student's capacity to follow the process of reflection, or is it the content of the reflection as an indication of the student's development in the specific competence area on which she is reflecting? Furthermore, because of the ubiquity of reflective assignments in many PA and other healthcare educational programs, students often find these multiple assignments burdensome and greet a new assignment with eye-rolling derision, eventually developing so-called reflection-fatigue. There is also no consensus in the medical education literature that reflection in healthcare education directly improves clinician's performance in practice or patient health outcomes.

Even accounting for these challenges, there is still much value in teaching and acquiring habits of reflection because of their benefits and compliment to other aspects of PA education.[11,12] Although a controversial stance in healthcare education, the author firmly believes that the process of reflection *can* be taught as a skill set and, with time, evolve into a set of effective habits of mind. The author even boldly asserts that this skill set can even be assessed, as long as what is being assessed is clearly defined—it is not the *content* of the reflection but the attainment of the *skills* associated with reflection.

It should be added that reflection, by itself, can be limited by the tendency of humans to be inaccurate when it comes to self-assessment. It has been determined conclusively that people are poor at self-assessment and that there is no way to learn or improve this ability. It is simply a reality that must be accepted.[13,14] Although reflection, even self-reflection, is not the same as self-assessment, it must be acknowledged that a PA cannot effectively judge his own abilities in any specific area of practice or a specific competence. The benefits of reflection are in its influence on our attitudes and affect—the openness to exploration of one's own habits and assumptions, gaining self-awareness and insight into one's own practices, and acknowledging our own challenges and barriers.

For a more robust approach to self-improvement, a PA student or practicing PA should combine habits of reflection with other sources of information on their individual performance; what Kevin Eva and Glenn Regehr refer to as "Self-Directed Assessment Seeking." They describe this as "a process by which one takes personal responsibility for looking outward, explicitly seeking feedback and information from external sources, then using these externally generated sources of assessment data to direct performance improvements. In this construction, self-assessment is more of a pedagogical strategy than an ability to judge for oneself; it is a habit that one needs to acquire and enact rather than an ability that one needs to master."[14 (p. 15)] Habit of self-reflection along with self-directed assessment-seeking habits would seem to be an ideal and complementary match.

SKILLS FOR REFLECTION

There is some debate about whether habits of reflection can or should be taught. The author strongly believe that habits of reflection are essential to PA practice, especially as they relate to the Professional role. They are integral components of life-long learning and self-improvement. Although some PAs may already possess related attributes or a tendency for reflective attitudes and behaviors, all PA should learn reflective habits of mind, as they learn pathophysiology or anatomy. An experienced reflective PA will eventually engage in this habit of mind subconsciously or automatically. However, reflection should be taught and assessed as a skill set in PA education.

For a beginner, it is helpful to use a structured format for reflection, even though the structure may be limiting in other ways. Just like in other contemplative or expressive activities, such as meditation or dance, the mechanics are the basis for effective expression. Mastering basic components and skills eventually allows opportunities for improvisation and free styling. This is also true of reflective habits.

The learning theorist David Kolb described four elements in the learning cycle: concrete experience; observation of, and reflection on, the experience; abstract conceptualization; and active experimentation. He explained that learning can begin at any of these stages but typically begins with a concrete experience.[15] Graham Gibbs, an education researcher, built on Kolb's learning cycle by developing a structured debriefing process, known as the Gibbs' Reflective Cycle.[16] This reflective cycle provides a useful starting point for the novice in developing reflective skills. Each step in this reflective cycle allows the PA to focus on specific components in her reflective toolbox.

As mentioned previously, although the process of reflection does not need to follow a specific order, it is helpful for a beginner to start with a reliable framework, such as Gibbs' Reflective Cycle. Starting with a framework enables one to think through the reflective process in an orderly fashion, with a beginning, middle, and end. It offers a nidus on which to attach the words evoked by the thoughts, feelings, and analysis of the process. Once the skills of reflection are ingrained, the order can be relaxed and steps skipped, as needed. Previously, we used dance or meditation as examples. Another way to think of it is following a recipe. Initially, especially for a complex dish, one should closely follow the recipe in a stepwise fashion. After a few tries, with some experience, the steps can be relaxed, ingredients can be added or left out, there is room for improvisation, and the final product will still be good, maybe even better.

Although there are several other reflective frameworks, the author chooses the Gibbs' Reflective Cycle[16] as a starting point, because of its relative simplicity, face validity, and completeness (*See Diagram at: https://www.brookes.ac.uk/students/ upgrade/study-skills/reflective-writing-gibbs/*).

FOLLOWING GIBBS' REFLECTIVE CYCLE

To begin with, the PA should consider a meaningful event or encounter on which to reflect. It could be a challenging patient encounter, a difficult team meeting, an event that triggered a strong emotion (either positive or negative), a medical error, an ethical dilemma, or a difficult clinical case that challenged the PA's knowledge or skills. The subject of reflection should be one that had a significant impact, as these are often the best situations from which to learn deeply and find meaning. Many students who learn the process of this reflective exercise are surprised by the depth of what they are able to analyze in their own practice. Many students, over the years, have expressed feeling of empowerment and even revelation when learning the process of reflection following the Gibbs' Reflective Cycle. They often compare it to a feeling such as exercising a muscle they did not know they had. It can be enlightening and impactful when PA students discover this new ability.

Now let us go through the cycle step by step. This can be done as a mental or written exercise. The advantage of writing is that it can be saved and used for later review. Sometimes the greatest impact of a reflective exercise occurs after the passage of time, with further delayed reflection. (We will avoid discussing reflecting on reflection, as this may induce severe eye-rolling.)

Stage 1: Description

The first step in the cycle is the description of the event. The PA will describe what happened in the encounter, in as much detail possible. Consider mainly objective aspects of the encounter and use many adjectives. The purpose in this section is to paint a picture with words. A more detailed description will evoke more of the thoughts and feeling for the next section and provide a richer foundation for the analysis to come. In this section, it is also helpful to try to leave out any *subjective* description. This is important because it is quite helpful in the reflection process to distinguish between objective and subjective experiences. For example, sometimes a student may describe an early patient encounter in which he struggled, by saying that the "room was spinning" or "time stood still." Although these both are extremely valuable observations, the student will often have a moment of realization when asked simple, seemingly obvious questions: *Was the room truly spinning? Did this encounter occur during an earthquake?* Or *Did the clock stop during the encounter? Was there some cosmic disruption in the progression of time?* Appreciating the subtle, yet significant, distinctions between objective and subjective experiences, even contrasting these, will help the PA make sense and build meaning in subsequent stages of the reflection. [a] In this stage, it is important not to draw conclusions or make judgments but simply to describe the event.

Stage 2: Thoughts and feelings

This section asks the PA to describe the subjective response to the encounter. The PA considers the following questions: *What thoughts were going through your mind? What emotions were coming to the surface? What was your gut-level reaction?* At this point, having described the scenario in rich objective language in the previous stage, the PA will be able to overlay thoughts and feelings onto this backdrop scenery. Because meaningful events will usually evoke a variety of thoughts and feelings, it is important to keep the scope of the encounter limited, by focusing on a short time duration or a specific part of an encounter. Often, the narrower the duration of the encounter, the deeper the reflection can dig. Again, this stage is for describing the subjective reaction, not for drawing conclusion or making judgments yet.

Stage 3: Evaluation

This section asks the PA to make a judgment about the event—what went well and what did not go well. This stage is short, acting as a pause and a transition to the analysis, which is at the heart of the reflective exercise.

Stage 4: Analysis

This is the meaty, meaning-making section of the reflective exercise. Having laid out the evidence provided by the objective description of the event and the subjective response of thoughts and feelings, the PA can begin to analyze these items; combine them; construct and deconstruct them; and relate them to other events, past experiences, or learned theories and phenomena.

The PA may discover that a certain feeling is associated with a specific event. For example, the PA may notice that she felt anxious when there was a silent gap in the conversation. This may have been the point when she felt that "time stood still." On further analysis, the PA may realize that she often feels anxious during periods of silence. This will give her more to analyze: Why does she feel anxious in these moments? Does she feel unprepared or unable to direct the patient encounter? Does the silence make her feel vulnerable or inexperienced? Or does she associate silence with negative emotions? Does she feel the need to fill the

---

[a] Some may argue that all experience is subjective. In describing the Gibbs' Reflection Cycle, the author uses the term *objective* to refer to those experiences that are perceived using the senses, in contract to cognitive or affective processes. For example, what did the room look like? How did the patient appear? What did the patient say? Was there a smell? etc.

void of silence by speaking? How can she develop the ability to tolerate silence, or even use it at appropriate times, for the purpose of building a therapeutic patient relationship?

This stage also encourages the PA to consider what they already know, such as any learning models or theories they have learned in the past that may relate to the event. Having a concrete experience can help with deeper understanding of a previously theoretic or abstract concept.

Stage 5: Conclusion

Like the Evaluation step, this section can be considered transitional. It asks the PA to draw conclusions about the experience and the analysis, so far. These conclusions may be general, or they can be specific and personal. The conclusion can be viewed as the summary of the previous analysis step.

Stage 6: Action Plan

Finally, and perhaps of greatest value in this process, the PA will determine a plan of action. The point of reflection is not simply to better understand our own actions and reactions in weighty situations. Rather, the purpose of reflection is to find a pathway to our better selves. If we can draw insights about ourselves, our behaviors, and our actions and reactions, we can consider ways to operationalize those insights into better ways of practicing, acting, and reacting in future similar situation. The key to creating a useful action plan is to follow the SMART acronym. Actions plans should be *S*pecific; *M*easurable; *A*chievable; *R*ealistic; and *T*imely.

This reflective process is a useful and powerful tool and can be used in many aspects of life, both professionally and personally. Once you go through the process several times in this (or another) formal stepwise approach, you may find that you begin to think reflectively at other times, as well, without the external prompt or the need to write down the steps of the cycle. The process itself begins to become tacit and implicit. You will be able to do it without explicit cognitive effort.

SUMMARY

Reflection is a higher-order metacognitive process that allows a PA to identify and analyze individual challenges in practice, with the purpose of addressing these challenges. The process of reflection allows the PA to develop actionable plans to address the gaps in current knowledge, skills, or attitudes.

Reflection is derived from the education psychology theories of reflective practice but has shifted from its theoretic foundations, to its common use in healthcare education and practice. Still, aspects of the theoretic framing can be applied to its common use. The concepts of reflection-in-action and reflection-on-action can inform the types of reflection a PA engages in—either in the moment, in the form of self-monitoring and making small, iterative adjustments, or after the event, considering challenging encounters, how and why they occurred, and how to better deal with a future similar encounter. Furthermore, reflection allows a PA to learn while *doing*—to address the real-world, complex challenges of clinical practice that can only be learned by *doing* them, not by learning *about* them.

Other benefits include nurturing of positive cognitive and affective habits, such as openness to feedback, a curiosity for self-exploration and self-awareness, and a desire for continued learning and professional development.

Although teaching and assessing reflection is a controversial topic, this article asserts that it is possible to teach the skills related to reflection, and to some degree, to assess them. It must be clear to students that it is only the process and skills acquisition that are being assessed, not the content; a reflection cannot be "wrong." In this article, the author describes one approach to reflection, following the steps of Gibbs' Reflective Cycle. Reflection lays the foundation for life-long learning and continued professional development. It is both a habit of mind and a skill set in which all PAs should be competent.

ACKNOWLEDGMENTS

The author would like to thank the Consortium of PA Education, the Department of Family & Community Medicine, and the University of Toronto for supporting the preparation of this article.

REFERENCES

1. Morton B. Falser words were never spoken - The New York Times, Opinion. The New York TImes 2011. Available at: https://www.nytimes.com/2011/08/30/opinion/falser-words-were-never-spoken.html. Accessed August 29, 2011.
2. Competencies for the physician assistant profession. JAAPA 2005;18(7):16–8. Available at: http://link.galegroup.com.myaccess.library.utoronto.ca/apps/doc/A160711804/AONE?u=utoronto_main&sid=AONE&xid=279e0ace.
3. Sandars J. The use of reflection in medical education: AMEE Guide No. 44. Med Teach 2009;31(8):685–95. Available at: https://www.ncbi.nlm.nih.gov/pubmed/19811204.
4. Jamieson KH. Letter from Joseph P Kennedy to Ted Sorensen, February 24, 1960, cited in AuthorPackaging the presidency: a history and criticism of presidential campaign advertising. New York: Oxford University Press; 1996.
5. Arseneau RR,D. The developmental perspective: cultivating ways of thinking. In: Pratt DD, editor. Five perspectives on teaching in adult and higher education. Malabar (FL): Krieger; 1998. p. 105–49.
6. Schön DA. Educating the reflective practitioner: toward a new design for teaching and learning in the professions. San Francisco (CA): Jossey-Bass; 1987.
7. Ng S. (2016). Re-imagining reflective practice in health professions education. Paper presented at the Best Practice in Education Rounds. Toronto, October 4, 2016.
8. Ng S. Reflection and reflective practice: creating knowledge through experience. Semin Hear 2012;33(02):117–34. Available at: https://www.thieme-connect.de/DOI/DOI?10.1055/s-0032-1311673.
9. Eva KW, Regehr G. Knowing when to look it up: a new conception of self-assessment ability. Acad Med 2007;82(10):S81–4. RIME: Proceedings of the Forty-Sixth Annual Conference November 4-November 7, 2007, Available at: https://ovidsp.ovid.com/ovidweb.cgi?T=JS&CSC=Y&NEWS=N&PAGE=fulltext&D=ovfti&AN=00001888-200710001-00022.
10. Moulton CAE, Regehr G, Mylopoulos M, et al. Slowing down when you should: a new model of expert judgment. Acad Med 2007;82(10):S109–16. RIME: Proceedings of the Forty-Sixth Annual Conference November 4-November 7, 2007, Available at: https://ovidsp.ovid.com/ovidweb.cgi?T=JS&CSC=Y&NEWS=N&PAGE=fulltext&D=ovfti&AN=00001888-200710001-00029.
11. Cavilla D. The effects of student reflection on academic performance and motivation. SAGE Open 2017;7(3). 2158244017733790. Available at: https://journals.sagepub.com/doi/abs/10.1177/2158244017733790.

12. Lew MDN, Schmidt HG. Self-reflection and academic performance: is there a relationship? Adv Health Sci Educ 2011;16(4):529.

13. Dunning D, Heath C, Suls JM. Flawed self-assessment: implications for health, education, and the workplace. Psychol Sci Public Interest 2004;5(3):69–106. Available at: http://www.jstor.org.myaccess.library.utoronto.ca/stable/40062350.

14. Eva KW, Regehr G. "I'll never play professional football" and other fallacies of self-assessment. J Contin Educ Health Prof 2008;28(1):14–9. Available at: http://resolver.scholarsportal.info/resolve/08941912/v28i0001/14_nppfaofos.

15. Kolb DA. Experiential learning: experience as the source of learning and development. 2nd edition. Upper Saddle River (NJ): Pearson Education, Inc; 2015.

16. Gibbs G. Learning by doing: a guide to teaching and learning methods. Further education unit. Oxford (United Kingdom): Oxford Polytechnic; 1988.

Practical Ethical Decision-Making for Physician Assistants

Sharona Kanofsky, PA-C, CCPA, MScCH

KEYWORDS

- Medical Ethics • Healthcare • Physician Assistant

KEY POINTS

- Physician Assistants (PAs) should be able to identify and respond to ethical dilemmas as soon as they arise in clinical and professional practice.
- PAs should appreciate and become proficient with the key principles that guide consideration and decision-making in cases of ethical dilemmas.
- An organized, stepwise approach is useful in addressing and resolving medical ethical dilemmas within a healthcare team.

INTRODUCTION

Ethical decision-making in healthcare is a critical skill set that all Physician Assistants (PAs) must learn. Although PAs often are not the most responsible provider in a medical team, they should not make the mistake of thinking they are absolved of difficult decisions. Ethical dilemmas, especially those that involve life-and-death decisions, are often made as a team. The PA's involvement can have significant impact, especially when the PA has the tools to help guide the decision-making process. Having a clear and thoughtful approach for considering and resolving ethical dilemmas arising in clinical and professional practice is an invaluable ability for any PA.

Ethical decisions can be big and small, life-altering or mundane, and occur regularly in clinical practice. PAs, as part of the healthcare team, will often be called on to express their thoughts and decision-making process on these tough choices, and they should be prepared.

An ethical dilemma is a question involving a moral or value-based decision that must be made, where there is potentially more than one possible course of action. An ethical dilemma challenges the healthcare provider to determine the *best* course of action

Department of Family and Community Medicine, Physician Assistant Program, 263 McCaul Street, 3rd Floor, Toronto, Ontario, M5T 1W7, Canada
E-mail address: sharona.kanofsky@utoronto.ca

Physician Assist Clin 5 (2020) 39–48
https://doi.org/10.1016/j.cpha.2019.08.004
2405-7991/20/© 2019 Elsevier Inc. All rights reserved.
physicianassistant.theclinics.com

among several possible options. However, there is usually no obvious "right" answer; each course of action may have advantages or disadvantages.

Ethics is a complex area within the greater field of Philosophy. Most PA and medical programs do not have the capacity to delve deeply into this field, and most health providers do not become experts unless they choose to specialize in this area. Still, PAs and other providers must be equipped with a practical skill set to address the ethical challenges that will surely arise in practice.

A PA must possess a basic set of skills to approach clinical ethical decision-making. These include the ability to clearly identify and articulate an ethical dilemma whenever one arises; a working facility with the basic ethical principles that guide clinical ethical decision-making; and a practical, reliable approach to decision-making.

IDENTIFYING AN ETHICAL DILEMMA

Identifying that an ethical dilemma exists may sound simple and obvious, but it often can be missed in the flurry of activities in the clinical setting. As PAs, we encounter many scenarios in clinical practice daily and most of them seem routine and expected. We have been trained to do the right thing with regularity: find out the issue that has motivated the patient to seek care; identify what is causing the problem; figure out a way to treat or manage the problem; and follow-up to make sure the patient is improving and feeling better. We try to do this all while ensuring we communicate well, interact with care and compassion, work effectively within the team, keep up to date with the best evidence, and so forth.

But what do we do when a situation is *uncertain*—when the *right* thing to do is not clear, obvious, or routine? The regular approach may not fit. The first things to consider are the following: *What is different about this scenario? Why did I stop to think? Why is this case not routine?* Is it a clinically difficult challenge? If so, it may require looking up the best practice guidelines or consulting with a supervising physician, another healthcare team member, or an outside expert. What if the challenge is not clinical, but rather a question about competing *values*? In this case, you have likely encountered an ethical dilemma. This is a good time to stop and name it—say to yourself "*I have an ethical dilemma.*" Once you have stopped yourself in your tracks, you will have a better chance of appropriately addressing, and hopefully resolving, this ethical challenge. Too often, clinicians miss this first step and miss the opportunity to approach an ethical challenge deliberately, using an organized approach. Only in retrospect is the ethical dilemma recognized. Clinicians can often trace these missed opportunities in hindsight to the exact moment when they should have stopped and recognized the ethical dilemma.

Sometimes, an ethical dilemma may not be addressed because it is perceived as common practice. It takes someone to notice a conflict of values or question standard practices—to see that what is considered normal is, in fact, ethically concerning. A prominent example is the once-common practice of medical trainees performing vaginal examinations on anesthetized women before gynecologic procedures. This was once considered an ideal opportunity for learners to practice vaginal examinations in a low-stress environment, while the patient is "asleep." Although many teaching hospitals request patient consent for learners to be involved in their care, these practice vaginal examinations were often not directly related to the woman's care; specific consent is required (and rarely obtained) to perform practice vaginal examinations. Still, the practice continued despite many learners feeling conflicted about doing it. It was deemed acceptable at one time, either because of the benefits to medical learning, and supposedly by extension, to the public, or because consent for these practice examinations was considered implicit. Finally, in 2007, a brave Canadian medical student questioned this practice and discovered how common it was; 72% of her peers had done practice vaginal examinations on unconscious patients, without obtained consent.[1] She later found that most women *do* expect to be asked specifically for consent *and* that most women would consent to students practicing, if asked in advance.[2] Soon after this, the Society of Obstetricians and Gynecologists of Canada revised its policy on this practice, and now explicit consent is required for this practice. Performing these examinations without specific consent is finally recognized as violations of personal autonomy, basic human rights, and trust between patients and providers,[3] yet it took a long time for this unethical practice even to be meaningfully questioned.

It is also important to be able to recognize when a question or choice to be made in practice is *not* an ethical dilemma. Often, especially for learners, the distinction may be unclear. A situation may be perceived as an ethical dilemma when it really is only a difficult choice or a clinical question—for example, deciding whether to perform a less invasive procedure that has a lower success rate or a riskier procedure with a higher success rate. This type of decision requires clinical consideration, weighing the extent of risks and benefits, the patient's input about preferences, and an appreciation of the patient's context, but it is not usually an ethical dilemma.

PRINCIPLES OF MEDICAL ETHICS

There are a few key principles in medical ethics that are used to frame and consider dilemmas and decision-making. These are usually referred to as the primary principles of autonomy; justice; and beneficence. Sometimes nonmaleficence is added to this list, as the first principle found in the Hippocratic Oath, *"Primum non nocere"* ("First do no harm"), although this principle can also be considered the alternate side of beneficence.

AUTONOMY

Autonomy relates to the primacy of each person's inalienable right to self-determination. In Western culture this is often considered the foremost of all the ethical principles—a sort of trump card. This guides every healthcare provider to respect the patient as the primary decision-maker in all personal health-related matters. Accordingly, the patient should always be given the required information to make an informed decision; the patient should always be told the results of any examination or investigation; and the patient's decisions about care and treatments should always be respected and followed, to the extent possible.

There are times when the patient is not able to communicate preferences and decisions, due to circumstances such as impaired cognition or physical incapacitation. At such times, the basic principle of autonomy remains intact. This means that the patient still holds the right to self-determination. The patient's wishes must be honored if the patient has made those wishes known in advance, either in writing or verbally. If not, the patient's preferences and wishes must be inferred through a designee, a substitute decision-maker (SDM). SDMs are responsible to infer the wishes of the patient as best as they can, from past communications, and with their familiarity with the patient's values and beliefs. The SDM is usually a close family member or life partner and usually has the background and insight to infer the patient's preferences. It must always be clear that an SDM is merely extending the patient's autonomy and not making decisions based on the SDM's own values and preferences. The role of the SDM can become complicated by the emotional attachment to a sick loved one. Acting as SDM is a serious responsibility, requiring a person to act dutifully as a true substitute for the patient and not making decision based on their own wishes or beliefs.

BENEFICENCE AND NONMALEFICENCE

The primary factor motivating most PAs who enter the profession in the first place is the desire to provide care for patients, ease their burden of illness, and provide the best path to health and wellness, that is, to benefit the patient using the tools of the PA trade. In resolving an ethical dilemma, the outcome that is most beneficial to the patient should be the goal. This can sometimes be challenging, as when the patient requests a treatment option that is not the most beneficial option, in your professional opinion, or when the patient refuses treatment that you deem beneficial. In this latter case, refusing treatment may, in your impression, harm the patient. The reason this poses a challenge is that we normally agree with our patients on what is beneficial and what is harmful. If an otherwise healthy patient has an uncomplicated fracture, the PA and the patient will typically agree that the most beneficial treatment is immobilization and pain management. However, there are times when a patient may decline treatment, such as at the end of life when they feel treatment will not improve their overall quality of life, or in severe mental illness when the patient is not motivated to get better. In such cases, the principles of autonomy and beneficence must be weighed. On one hand, we respect the patient's right to determine and guide their own care. On the other hand, we are responsible to ensure that the outcome is the most beneficial one to the patient, even when it means the patient determines what is beneficial, not the healthcare team. Of course, the question of capacity must be addressed to ensure that the patient is making informed decisions, as will be discussed shortly.

JUSTICE

The principle of justice assumes that each person is entitled to a fair share of healthcare resources. No person should be entitled to better or more care that another, based on their social or economic status, or any other factor. At the same time, there are limits to how far one person's entitlement can go. The benefit of one person may interfere with the wellbeing of others, such as when the safety of others is in question, or with allocation of limited shared resources.

This principle of justice acknowledges the hard truth that there is a limit to healthcare resources, such as money, equipment, and human resources. There is a societal lens to ethical decision-making that must consider the contextual reality in which ethical dilemmas are resolved. These cases often attract massive media attention because they involve some of the hardest questions in healthcare, such as, *When has a person reached the limit of what is considered just and fair allocation of healthcare resources?* The patient's SDMs often argue stridently that the benefit of keeping their loved one alive, even mechanically, and the over-riding principle of autonomy—the right of the SDM to determine care on the patient's behalf—override the ability of the legal or institutional decision-makers to "pull the plug" for the practical concerns of resource allocation. Some of the toughest cases occur in real situations where resources, such as mechanical ventilators in neonatal care units, must be triaged to the patients who can most benefit from them. The principle of justice echoes the common utilitarian axiom, "the greatest good for the greatest number."

TELLING THE TRUTH

A common question related to patient autonomy is whether or not to tell a patient the truth about the medical prognosis. Respecting a patient's right to self-determination implies a responsibility to provide all health-related information; as the courtroom expression goes, "The truth, the whole truth, and nothing but the truth." There has been a shift in attitudes regarding truth telling over the past few decades.[4] It was once considered cruel to tell patients, for example, that they had a terminal illness. It was even considered detrimental to their health to divulge that they may have only a limited time to live. The news of physical and existential suffering and the expected loss of hope that would result were considered too difficult to bear and therefor harmful. To be sure, there are still significant cultural and personal variations in patients' attitudes to what they want to hear from their medical team. However, the trends have shifted significantly in this area. Patients now often want to know the truth and believe that they can handle it.[5] There is a new appreciation that knowing the truth helps patients develop trust in their healthcare providers and family members and that there are additional benefits related to closure, emotional and logistical preparation, reconciliation, and personal reflection when patients know they are at the end of life.[6]

CONSENT

Informed consent, also called informed choice or informed decision-making,[7] is primarily a protection extended to patients. It ensures that any medical intervention is provided with the patient's free will, and with sufficient information to make the best decisions, from the patient's perspective. Consent is predicated on the assumptions of autonomy—that patients have the right to make their own health decisions, even if they are unpopular or ill-advised. This is true, as long as the patient has the cognitive capacity to make the decision, and it will not cause harm to others. Informed consent discourages attitudes of paternalism and authoritarianism in physicians, PAs, and other health providers involved in supporting patient decision-making.

The information that is required to communicate includes anything that will help the patient make an informed choice about the procedure or intervention. This includes the details of the intervention; the expected outcomes; possible alternatives to treatment; risks, such as possible side effects and adverse events; potential benefits of the intervention; and relative risks and benefits compared with alternative interventions, including the option of no intervention at all. Health information can be confusing and overwhelming to patients and loved ones, especially when facing major health issues. Communication around informed decision-making may take time and may require more than one conversation. It is the responsibility of the healthcare team to ensure that the patient has received and has understood all the relevant information to make the best choice for the patient.

Although informed consent also offers protection against litigation to healthcare providers, especially with appropriate documentation of the process, this is not the primary purpose of communicating with the patient and obtaining consent. The protection afforded clinicians by obtaining and documenting informed consent exists only because it is the right thing to do in the first place. It is important to remember that the primary purpose of obtaining a patient's consent is to uphold the ethical values underpinning autonomy and the right to self-determination, not to protect clinicians against litigation. With this view, emphasis can rightly be placed on patient-centered decision-making and good communication, ensuring the patient has the information needed, rather than ensuring the clinician has provided the minimum required information to check the boxes and secure legal protection.

CAPACITY

Although the basic ethical principles of autonomy and self-determination protect the right to make decisions about one's own medical care, there are limits to this right. If a person's decision will lead to harm or risk to others, this right does not extend that far. For example, a person may choose to smoke despite the known health risks; however, the person cannot expose others to airborne toxins by smoking in a smoke-free zone.

Generally, the principles of medical ethics protect a person's right to make decisions, even bad ones. The perspective is key—we may consider a bad decision something that will increase a person's risk of illness or death, but the patient may not see it that way. A person may prefer the momentary pleasure of a risky or unhealthy behavior to the long-term benefits of abstinence or may just be more risk-tolerant than a more risk-averse friend or PA. A so-called bad decision in the PA's judgment may be a good decision from the patient's perspective. This may be one of the most challenging aspects in providing care; allowing a patient to make a choice with which we do not agree. It is difficult to resist the reflex to impose our own judgment of what is best, when the patient does not want our "best" treatment option. All this is true as long as the patient has the capacity to make an informed choice, and that choice does not impinge on the autonomy or wellbeing of another.

It may seem obvious that a person's right to self-determination ends where a safety risk to another person begins, as in the smoking example discussed earlier. The question is more complex when determining whether to honor a person's healthcare decisions if it will lead to harm only to that person and not to others. When is it appropriate to protect a person from himself?

Capacity determines a person's ability to make a rational and unimpaired decision. As mentioned previously, people have the right to make health-related decisions that are considered "bad" by the healthcare team members. However, in the case of cognitive impairment, a patient may be unable to make an informed decision. In these cases, the healthcare professionals may need to override the patient's decision to protect the patient. This must be done cautiously, sometimes reluctantly, because of the high value placed on patient autonomy.

There are several vulnerable populations in which the question of capacity commonly arises. Children do not necessarily have the maturity and insight to grasp the weight and consequences of their actions. For example, cases of children going on hunger strikes in political protest raise the question of whether these children have the ability to rationally and freely make the choice to starve themselves or whether this is considered child abuse and the children should be force-fed to protect and save them.[8]

Children, however, do have some degree of insight and ability to understand the consequences of their decisions. This ability generally increases with age. But regardless of age, capacity in children must be considered in the context of the decision to be made. A young child may refuse an immunization, thinking only of the immediate pain associated with the injection. Healthcare staff and parents regularly use various forms of cajoling, distractions, bribery, and even physical restraint, to complete the child's immunization schedule. This common practice relies on the assumption that the child does not have the insight or the capacity to appreciate that the benefits of immunization far outweigh the momentary discomfort of the procedure. The assumption is that if the child had that insight—if she were her adult self looking backwards in time—she would surely agree to the procedure. To illustrate the point that capacity and consent in children is relative, depending on context and situation, some jurisdictions, such as Ontario, have no legal minimum age for consent.

Another vulnerable population, when it comes to consent and protection against self, are patients with progressive dementia, such as Alzheimer disease or vascular dementia. Although the ideal is to maintain these patients' right to autonomous health-related decisions, it is not always clear the extent to which they have the capacity to make these decisions in an informed way. Similar to the case with children, patients with dementia have the capacity to make some decisions, depending on context and situation. What further complicates the issue in this specific population is that cognitive abilities, and therefore capacity, can wax and wane in dementia. For example, for many patients in the middle stages of Alzheimer, there is an increase in confusion at the end of the day, commonly referred to as sundowning. Such a patient may have a clearer ability to make a decision in the early part of the day but may lose that ability in the evenings. At times, there is no predictable pattern to the peaks and valleys in mental clarity, confounding the PA's ability to determine if a health-related decision is made insightfully or if the patient lacks the capacity to make that particular decision at that particular moment.

A third vulnerable population is patients with mental or emotional disorders. These cases can also be tricky because there is no clear line delineating what degree of mental or emotional instability renders a person incapable of making an informed choice. As in young age and progressive dementia, capacity tends to fluctuate or depend on context in patients with psychiatric illness.

In a famous case from the 1970s, Dax Cowart was a patient who suffered severe burns over most of his body in an accidental explosion.[9] Throughout his excruciating treatment, he repeatedly requested that his treatment be stopped and that he be allowed to die. Nevertheless, his treatments continued, and after many surgeries and painful treatments, he survived, with severe physical disabilities, including blindness. Eventually, he became a lawyer and patients-rights advocate. One of the reasons his healthcare team ignored his wishes to stop treatment was that they considered him incapable of making informed decisions about his care. They maintained that he did not have the capacity due to the influence of medications and severe pain, which they believed clouded his judgment, despite a psychiatric assessment that determined that he was, in fact, competent. This story illustrates that physical, psychiatric, or existential distress do not always render a patient incapable of decision-making, even in extreme situations.

A DECISION-MAKING PROCESS

Ethical dilemmas, by definition, do not lend themselves to simple answers. There are no algorithms, guidelines, or equations that can be readily applied to tell you the right thing to do. Usually there are conflicting principles at play. Patient autonomy must be weighed against public safety in the case of a patient with dementia who wishes to live independently, despite the potential danger of unwittingly causing a kitchen fire. In the case of a patient demanding antibiotic treatment of a likely viral respiratory infection, societal risks of overprescribing antibiotics must be weighed against the patient's autonomy. There are often several possible courses of action to address an ethical dilemma, but each option still leaves part of the dilemma unresolved. The PA, as part of the healthcare team, is responsible to determine the *best* possible course of action that *best* satisfies at least some of the issues.

The challenges in resolving ethical dilemmas call for an organized approach, whereby the healthcare teams can follow a reliable process to address most ethical dilemmas they will encounter. Dr Philip Hébert outlines just such a stepwise decision-making approach in his book, *Doing Right: A Practical Guide to Ethics for Medical Trainees and Physicians*. [10(pp14–18)]

According to Dr Hebert, the first step in addressing an ethical dilemma is recognizing that one exists in the first place, as discussed earlier. Many ethical challenges that PA students have shared with the author from their clinical training were complicated by the fact that they were not recognized early. It is imperative to stop and *notice* that an ethical dilemma has presented itself as soon as possible. This may take the form of questioning a previously accepted practice, as illustrated previously. The second step in the process is to articulate the ethical dilemma. In one *Ethics* course in a Canadian PA Program, the author found that even though students may recognize that something is "wrong," sometimes just at the gut level, they often struggle to articulate exactly what the ethical dilemma is. Clearly defining an ethical dilemma is crucial to meaningfully approach and consider the possible solutions, and to eventually arrive at a resolution. Often, it is helpful to formulate the ethical question using a variation of the formulation, "*In the case of Patient X, should alternative Y occur?*" For example, *In the case of a 75-year-old woman with advanced dementia and diabetes, should a leg amputation be performed?*

The third step involves laying out possible alternatives. This process requires the PA to think of as many courses of action as possible. At first, the novice may think the choices are binary: continue mechanical ventilation or discontinue; perform the surgery or do not perform the surgery; tell the parents that the teenage daughter is requesting birth control or do not tell them. However, there often is a third or fourth reasonable alternative to consider. Sometimes, these additional alternatives are compromises "in between" the *do or do not* spectrum of options. At other times, especially with some creative thinking, the third or fourth alternative adds an option entirely new to the equation, a novel approach that had not previously been considered. One example is introducing the option to wait and defer the decision for a prescribed period of time; with some perspective and time to reflect, decisions can become clearer.

Creative solutions can be refreshing and enlightening; sometimes the best solutions to get unstuck from a seemingly uncompromising dilemma come from thinking outside the box. For example, consider two adult children who are trying to convince their widowed father to move from his townhouse home of 50 years into a nursing home. Lately, he has become forgetful. There was a recent scare involving leaving a stove burner on all night. The father adamantly refuses to move to the nursing home, but his children fear for his safety and that of the neighbors. They get locked in a power struggle over his right to decide for himself where to live versus the safety issues. Eventually, a thoughtful PA inquires about the family's resources and discovers that one of the siblings has the space in her home to comfortably accommodate the father. The father is amenable to this arrangement and is able to employ a part-time caregiver with his retirement savings and money from the sale of his house. No one had previously considered this arrangement, but everyone is pleased. The father is relieved to move in with his daughter, instead of into a nursing home. It emerges that he was also concerned about his declining memory and related safety issues, but he felt too defensive to admit this when feeling threatened with institutionalization. The adult children are both relieved that their father will be comfortable and properly looked after. This is an example of effective out-of-the-box practical ethical decision-making.

The fourth step involves weighing the options using the ethical principles. One alternative solution may favor the patient's autonomy, whereas another may seem more just, from the perspective of the healthcare system. One alternative may seem more beneficial than another. This step is critical in comparing the pros and cons of each possible alternative solution, based on the ethical principles and how they are applied in the case. This weighting exercise will usually lead to the best alternative.

The fifth step asks the clinician to consider who else should be involved in the decision, if not already involved. This could be another specialist, a social worker or mental health professional, another healthcare professional, clinical ethicist, family member, spiritual counselor, or a designated ombudsperson. This step also asks the clinician to consider contextual factors that may not have been attended to yet, such as relevant laws and policies, or the emotional state of the patient.

The sixth step is to choose the best option, having weighed all the options against one another, considered the ethical principles, consulted with others, as appropriate, and considered contextual factors. There often will not be a perfect solution; if there was, there likely would be no dilemma to begin with. However, the *best* choice is one with which the patient will hopefully feel satisfied and that will allow the clinical team to sleep well at night, knowing they have done the best they can in the situation.

The seventh step is to review and reconsider the decision critically and ensure that nothing was missed, and all factors were considered. Some questions to ask yourself include the following: *Under what circumstances might my decision be different?* and *Is this decision realistic and practically doable?* The final step is to *act* based on the decision made. This may seem obvious, but it takes the decision-making process from abstraction to action. This is also when the clinician can feel the tension, as well as the satisfaction, of doing something that may be difficult, but which is ultimately *right*, in the sense of being the *best* solution to a difficult dilemma.[10]

SUMMARY

Ethical decision-making is an important area of competence for PAs. Both the American and Canadian PA competency frameworks include ethical decision-making in the professional role/domain. [11(p3, pp21,22),12] Ethical dilemmas in clinical practice are some of the most challenging moments for any PA. Many day-to-day clinical challenges lend themselves more readily to right and wrong solutions. The results of clinical decisions often reveal themselves to be correct, or not, by favorable or unfavorable health outcomes. By contrast, ethical decisions do not often offer clear and easy solutions nor does the outcome readily lend itself to retrospective validation of the decisions made. They are called dilemmas precisely because there are no clear or easy answers.

To gain competence in ethical decision-making, a PA should be able to identify and clearly articulate an ethical dilemma as soon as it arises, proficiently and sensitively apply the principles of medical ethics, and follow an organized, stepwise approach to resolving the ethical dilemma, as part of the healthcare team. Having applied these skills competently, a PA and her team can feel satisfied, knowing that they have arrived at the best possible solution to a difficult ethical challenge.

ACKNOWLEDGMENTS

The author would like to thank the Consortium of PA Education, the Department of Family & Community Medicine, and the University of Toronto for supporting the preparation of this article. The author would also like to thank Dr. Philip Hébert for his ongoing guidance and support over the years.

REFERENCES

1. Picard A. Time to end pelvic exams done without consent. The globe and mail. 2010. Available at: https://www.theglobeandmail.com/life/health-

and-fitness/time-to-end-pelvic-exams-done-without-consent/article4325965/. Accessed January 8, 2010.

2. Chamberlain S, Bocking A, McGrath M, et al. Teaching pelvic examinations under anaesthesia: what do women think?. Available at: http://ovidsp.ovid.com/ovidweb.cgi?T=JS&CSC=Y&NEWS=N&PAGE=fulltext&D=med6&AN=20677393. Accessed February 5, 2019.

3. Friesen P. Educational pelvic exams on anesthetized women: Why consent matters. Bioethics 2018;32(5):298–307. Available at: http://ovidsp.ovid.com/ovidweb.cgi?T=JS&CSC=Y&NEWS=N&PAGE=fulltext&D=prem&AN=29687469.

4. Ruhnke GW, Wilson SR, Akamatsu T, et al. Ethical decision making and patient autonomy: a comparison of physicians and patients in Japan and the United States. Available at: http://ovidsp.ovid.com/ovidweb.cgi?T=JS&CSC=Y&NEWS=N&PAGE=fulltext&D=med4&AN=11035693. Accessed February 5, 2019.

5. Kirk P, Kirk I, Kristjanson LJ. What do patients receiving palliative care for cancer and their families want to be told? A Canadian and Australian qualitative study. BMJ 2004;328(7452):1343. Available at: https://www.bmj.com/content/bmj/328/7452/1343.full.pdf.

6. Tuckett A. Truth-telling in clinical practice and the arguments for and against: a review of the literature. Nurs Ethics 2004;11(5):500–13. Available at: http://resolver.scholarsportal.info/resolve/09697330/v11i0005/500_ticpataarotl.

7. Braddock CH III, Edwards KA, Hasenberg NM, et al. Informed decision making in outpatient practicetime to get back to basics. JAMA 1999;282(24):2313–20.

8. Mok A, Nelson EAS, Murphy J, et al. Children on hunger strike: child abuse or legitimate protest? Br Med J 1996;312(7029):501–4. Available at: http://www.jstor.org.myaccess.library.utoronto.ca/stable/29730764.

9. Pasquella D. Dax's Case. New York: Concern for Dying; 1984.

10. Hebert PC. Doing right: a practical guide to ethics for medical trainees and physicians. 3rd edition. Don Mills (Ontario): Oxford University Press; 2014.

11. Competencies for the Physician Assistant Profession. 2012. Available at: https://prodcmsstoragesa.blob.core.windows.net/uploads/files/PACompetencies.pdf. Accessed December 5, 2019.

12. CanMEDS-PA. Ottawa (Ontario): Canadian Association of Physician Assistants; 2015. Available at. https://capa-acam.ca/wp-content/uploads/2015/11/CanMEDS-PA.pdf.

Communication Considerations for Physician Assistants

Using Knowledge, Exploring Content, Following Process, and Heightening Perceptions

Maureen Gottesman, MD, MEd, CCFP[a,b,*]

KEYWORDS

- Communication • Knowledge • Content • Process • Perception
- Physician Assistants

KEY POINTS

- The role of communicator is one of the intrinsic attributes for physician assistants.
- The complexities of communication can be discussed in a framework that compartmentalizes various aspects.
- The knowledge of what types of communication are to be used in which circumstances (and why), the content of what is to be communicated, the process of how to communicate and the perceptions of internal realizations should be taken collectively, as the sum is greater than each of the parts.

INTRODUCTION

Effective communication is essential in all human relationships. This is especially true in the healthcare field. Medical providers of care are responsible to gather health information to apply clinical reasoning toward diagnosis and eventual management of the health of patients. Physician Assistants (PAs), as extenders of the supervising physicians and as part of practice teams, play an essential role in the effective gathering of patient information. PAs are entrusted to convey this information in the appropriate

Disclosure Statement: The author has no commercial nor financial conflicts of interest to declare. The author has not received any funding for this work.

a Department of Family and Community Medicine, Faculty of Medicine, University of Toronto, 263 McCaul Street, 3rd Floor, Toronto, Ontario M5T 1W7, Canada; b Department of Family and Community Medicine, North York General Hospital, Toronto, Ontario, Canada
* Department of Family and Community Medicine, Faculty of Medicine, University of Toronto, 263 McCaul Street, 3rd Floor, Toronto, Ontario M5T 1W7, Canada.
E-mail address: m.gottesman@utoronto.ca
Twitter: @maureengottesma (M.G.)

Physician Assist Clin 5 (2020) 49–60
https://doi.org/10.1016/j.cpha.2019.08.006

manner, informing the healthcare team, documenting data in the medical records, and educating patients.

This article explores the various elements of effective communication as an intrinsic skill and series of competencies that are instrumental in being a competent, practicing PA. The skills used to communicate, what is being communicated, and how, are outlined. One's own role as a partner in communication is explored.

As will be uncovered in the exploration of the intrinsic skills that make up the role of communicator, understanding the context of oneself and that of the partner(s) in communication are important. As such, the reader should appreciate the context of this author. As a founding medical/program director for one of the Canadian PA education programs, this author developed and implemented the clinical skills curriculum with the rest of the faculty team. Civilian PA schools in Canada are affiliated with Faculties of Medicine and use medical school principles and methods to educate the PA learners. Communication skills are a fundamental part of PA education, and the key and enabling competencies developed over the course of PA school and along the practice continuum, as clinicians gain more experience and practice.

CONTENT

The communicator role is one of seven that is outlined in CanMEDS-PA[1] (medical expert, communicator, collaborator, leader, health advocate, scholar, and professional), the blue print modified from medical school education and used in PA education in Canada. These seven roles help to define the competencies of practicing PAs in Canada and are used to develop training and assessments for the national profession. Communication is a complex concept. The role of communicator in the context of PA competencies is described as, "...PAs effectively facilitate patient-centered care and the dynamic exchanges that occur before, during, and after the medical encounter."[1] The skill of communication itself has been defined as a "2-way process" aimed to transmit and share information to "create a shared interpretation" between those involved.[2,3] To better unpack the complexities of communication and apply it to the PA profession, a framework published in a recent systematic review is most suitable. This review identifies and categorizes a comprehensive list of communication skills, using learning outcomes, based on work collated from across the health professions education research.[3] Denniston and colleagues[3] compiled a list of 205 communication skills that are organized into four domains that provide a framework for exploring communication for healthcare professionals. The four domains according to Denniston et al are:

"1. Knowledge (eg, describe the importance of communication in healthcare)
2. Content skills (eg, explore a healthcare seeker's motivation for seeking healthcare)
3. Process skills (eg, respond promptly to a communication partner's questions)
4. Perceptual skills (eg, reflect on own ways of expressing emotion)."

The complexities of communication skills are not unique to any one profession. This article highlights and summarizes some key elements to communication that affect both PA students and PAs in clinical practice. Using the framework of Denniston and colleagues,[3] these four domains are explored in more detail: each domain will include a table of subcategories, quoting from their published work, and a selection, paraphrased, from their 205 published learning outcomes that are most relevant to PA communication in practice. Narrative and practical applications are organized by the domains that follow.

Knowledge (Knowing About Communication)

Breaking down the complexity of communication into its fundamental parts can help a PA acquire competence in this domain. Understanding the *what* about communication, meaning *what* is communication all about, has been identified as an important step in developing the overall competence. This means that it is not enough to follow the steps taught in communication skills but one must have an understanding of why these skills are important and effective. Similarly, one develops a professional identity and sense of professionalism by learning what the profession is all about, what it means to act professionally in practice. One develops the ability to be a skilled communicator by learning about communication in detail. PAs are part of the health-care team and do not work in isolation. Understanding the roles and responsibilities of other members of the team allows the PA to ensure they are working efficiently, effectively and collaboratively, as part of that team.

Physician assistant communication with patients

To develop communication skills, it is imperative to understand the purpose of these skills. When interviewing a patient, using patient-centered communication has been proven to enhance patient satisfaction, increase patient compliance, and, likely enables patients to achieve better outcomes.[4] "Telling" a patient that he or she should just stop smoking is not effective. "Counseling" for smoking cessation is far more effective, if done in a patient-centered way. What is meant by "counseling" is a series of subskills that are developed over time by the clinician and include specific interviewing techniques, such as active listening, assessing ambivalence and resistance to change, and negotiating a plan with the patient's priorities, values, and context at the forefront. An understanding of why these interview techniques are important is vital to developing the skill. Learned communication skills in the context of patient encounters can be applied to other situations as well.

Physician assistant communication with supervising physicians

The scope of practice of a PA is defined by the scope of practice of their supervising physician. Thus, the communication between the PA and physician is one of the most essential elements to be an effective healthcare provider (for both parties!). The nature of the communication may change over time, as the relationship evolves, and trust and scope of practice develop.

PAs are uniquely positioned at the front-line in gathering the clinical information from the patient. Depending on the level of autonomy, the PA may be expected to communicate that health information to the supervising physician. The ability to be thorough yet succinct, accurate yet organized and nonjudgmental, while using clinical reasoning to develop an assessment and plan, are all essential elements of communication.

Physician assistant communications with members of the healthcare team

PAs are responsible not only to their patients and their supervising physician, but to other members of the healthcare team. In the province of Ontario, Canada, where the PA profession is not yet regulated, there may be practical implications of this interaction. For the sake of this discussion, the PA may be working under a restricted scope in which basic clinical practice is confined. As an example, patient orders or prescriptions written by the PA may need to be cosigned by their supervising physician. Patients may need to be assessed by the physician, even after the PA assessment, to allow the physician to bill for the services rendered (and thus to pay the PA). These limitations are due to the regulated restrictions in the jurisdiction. However, for PAs working in well-functioning teams, which includes effective communication among the team members, many of these limitations can be overcome. The local pharmacists that meet the PA and are familiar with the clinical practice of the supervising physician may accept the prescription without a physician signature (often with a reference on the prescription to the relevant medical directive). Communication among team members may help to overcome some logistical barriers.

Physician assistant communication with the public
As part of the emerging PA profession in Canada, PAs are under scrutiny in the eyes of the public. It is incumbent on PAs to maintain a level of professionalism and integrity that the public will respect and admire. This includes interactions with the public or with an individual in a public forum, with supervising physicians, managers, hospital administrators, and other professionals and members of government.

Physician assistant communications and the medical record
PAs are expected to document in the medical record, yet understanding what to document (and how, covered in the content domain) is essential. For example, the PA may uncover much data in the course of a patient encounter. The PA's job is to filter and prioritize the order and content of what to include in the documentation. Sometimes, the profession of the patient is a key element that should be at the forefront (eg, "35-year-old pilot with a painful swollen leg" or "55-year-old firefighter with chronic cough"), and sometimes it would be irrelevant. Sometimes the chief complaint does not correspond with the most important issue that has arisen in the patient interaction: For example, "75-year-old man with a history of alcoholism presents with abdominal pain and episodes of vomiting blood." The 75-year-old may have come in because of the pain, and only on questioning would reveal the current overuse of alcohol. Only with effective communication skills would the PA be able to identify that the patient may have serious esophageal varices or other life-threatening causes of upper gastrointestinal bleeding. While conducting the interview, the PA demonstrates effective verbal and nonverbal communication skills to enable the patient to feel safe and share the story in a nonjudgmental environment. The PA is expected to develop rapport with the patient and attempt to understand the patient's context. The information that is documented leaves the data for future reference and must remain nonjudgmental and respectful.

The PA is responsible for understanding how communication expectations may be different under various circumstances. Slowing the pace, talking directly to the patient, and increasing eye contact when interviewing a patient with the help of an interpreter will enhance the patient-centered experience. Understanding the reporting, contact tracing and documentation expectations in a specific jurisdiction when dealing with sensitive issues, such as sexually transmitted infections, is vital not only for professional competence, but also to comply with legal requirements and to maintain the ongoing privacy of the patient.

Denniston and colleagues[3] break down the "knowledge" of communication into five subdomains listed in **Table 1**. Their work summarizes published numerous learning outcomes on communication skills from health professions education. Learning outcomes are statements that are specific and measurable. They include action verbs that can be observed and assessed by others. A sample from their learning outcomes is paraphrased here, selected from their comprehensive list. These were selected for this article as the most relatable to the essential communication skills for PAs in professional practice.

Table 1
Knowledge of communication: subdomains and selected learning outcomes

Knowledge[3] of Communication: Subdomains	Examples of Learning Outcomes[3] in This Domain (*As a Practicing PA, I Can…*)
"Purposes of communication in healthcare"	• Define barriers to communication • Recognize strengths and limitations when communicating in healthcare • Describe patient-centered communication • Define interprofessional relationships and teamwork
"Characteristics of communication"	• Describe the purpose of written and verbal communication, including documentation • Describe the use of nonverbal communication • Discuss types of communication skills used for patient interactions, such as open-ended and closed-ended questions, behavior change, and motivational interviewing
"Relationships and communication"	• Describe how rapport can be established in a communication encounter • Identify factors (such as power imbalance, personal context) that can impact the communication dynamic with others
"Emotions and communication"	• Describe challenges in having difficult conversations and the skills are required for these types of conversations • Define empathy and how is it demonstrated • Explain how thoughts and feelings can impact one's communication with others
"Communication modes"	• Recognize common short forms and acceptable abbreviations in the healthcare settings • Describe the reporting and documentation requirements by law in the setting and jurisdiction of clinical practice • Describe essential communication skills to enable successful interactions when working with interpreters

Content (What Is It That Needs to Be Communicated)

The content of communication seems the most obvious of the domains. It is the basic breakdown of what is required for the healthcare provider to ascertain from the patient, teammate, colleague, and so forth. There are countless guides, templates, mnemonics, and resources on *what* is required in various situations.

The content domain can be broken down into many detailed subdomains, starting with the physical space and introductions. The nonverbal behavior of how the clinician interacts with the physical space to ensure patient comfort, dignity, and privacy is a powerful set of communication tools that will also affect the rapport. For those communities less familiar with the PA profession, it behooves the PA to use the encounter as an opportunity to educate and clarify roles, not only to patients, but to others in the healthcare team, patient families, and the public, depending on the context.

The structure for the clinical encounter is the simplest way to explain what the content domain of communication is all about. One of the most common formats to document a follow-up clinical encounter is the "SOAP" progress note. This format provides a structure to document the encounter that would generally occur in a specific order: "Subjective" (meaning the patient's version of what is going on); "Objective" (meaning the healthcare provider's physical examination and other objective metrics, such as laboratory test results); "Assessment" (meaning the impression or diagnosis based on the collected information); and "Plan" (meaning the management steps, follow-up, and other action items). The communication skill of learning how to document a SOAP note, however, is more than simply regurgitating what the patient said and what occurred, in sequential order. When taken in context of the previous domain of knowledge, the intrinsic ability to be an effective communicator can be realized. Knowing which parts of the patient's story are most relevant, where to put these in the written note, and in what order, are prime examples of looking at communication skills as much greater than the sum of the individual parts.

Patients may present with a concern, and through skilled communication, more relevant information may lead the PA to realize that the main issue is more serious than the chief concern may have seemed. For example, the pilot with the sore leg may have been concerned about using up sick days at work and not being able to fly; however, once gathering the information, assessing risk factors, and completing a physical examination, the PA may be more concerned with a possible deep vein thrombosis and the pilot's risk for developing a pulmonary embolus, or a stroke, both of which may not have been on the patient's agenda at all. Using an established structure to the communication encounter while exploring the concerns of the patient contributes to optimal care.

The previous example of mentioning the patient's profession early in the medical document can be explored further. Including the patient's profession, psychosocial situation, family history, and other seemingly "nonmedical" details may all be included in the context of a clinical encounter if those details are seen to be clinically relevant. Of course, understanding the patient holistically can be the justification in many situations. However, when practicing medicine in resource restricted, time-constrained environments, healthcare providers, including PAs, may not always have the luxury to "get to know" their patient to such depths. Nonetheless, it can always be justified, and is often vital, to understand the patient's context.

Context and perspective assume even greater importance when dealing with conflict and difficult conversations. Discussing end-of-life wishes and goals of care are often seen as difficult conversations for most clinicians. Families that are unsatisfied with the care of their loved one can present as a conflict waiting to explode. Strategies to assist in overcoming these difficult situations stem from exploring the context of the communication partner. Exploring the values, religious or spiritual beliefs, and past experiences are fundamentally important before asking about resuscitation wishes from a family of a patient at the end of life. Investigating the concerns of a family, identifying their expectations for care, and the mismatch about expectations provided are part of the approach of dealing with conflict. However, exploring the context of those complaining are equally valid. Perhaps they had similar experiences in the past with negative outcomes, so they are simply trying to prevent a repeat episode. Perhaps they have a financial burden to which the current care plan is simply adding. Exploring context is fundamental to avoiding conflict.

PAs may find themselves in a position to offer patients recommendations, counseling, and management plans. As such, the clinician should have the communication skills to effectively convey information, guide patients toward behavior change, and motivate healthcare seekers to follow agreed-on advice. PAs are in the position to discuss informed consent with patients and must ensure they are familiar with the aspects of consent, including explaining the associated material risks and benefits.

Closing a communication encounter should not be rushed. Patients and other communication partners should be given the opportunity to clarify or ask outstanding questions, or, if time does not allow, there must be clear follow-up arrangements including on how to best contact each other. Beyond the patient encounter, PAs should have a clear plan with physician supervisors about how and when to be in contact if and when the need may arise.

Table 2 streamlines the "Content" of communication into 12 subdomains with related examples of learning outcomes.

Table 2
Content of communication: subdomains and selected learning outcomes

Content[3] of Communication: Subdomains	Examples of Learning Outcomes[3] in This Domain (*As a Practicing PA, I Can…*)
"Physical space"	• Ask permission to enter physical space with patients • Use physical tools like curtains, sheets, doors to respect privacy of others and maintain comfort of others when possible
"Opening and introductions"	• Introduce self and role • Clarify how the patient would like to be addressed
"Structure"	• Gather relevant information from multiple sources if available • Guide the patient interaction with logical flow from beginning to end • Collaborate with healthcare seeker to prioritize the agenda • Ask permission to progress with the encounter through various stages and signpost through these stages (history topics, physical examination, diagnosis, plan)
"Explore concerns"	• Explore the concerns of the health seeker and their motivation for seeking care at this time • Identify concerns that can be physical, emotional, and psychological
"Perspective"	• Acknowledge the perspective of the communication partner • Work toward a shared understanding
"Contextual factors"	• Explore the personal context of the healthcare seeker • Identify the various psychosocial factors of the healthcare seeker in relevance to their presenting issues
"Diagnosis"	• Provide diagnosis in relation to the presenting issue • Assess the health seeker's readiness to hear the diagnosis • Explain prognosis in context of diagnosis as realistically as possible
"Decision making"	• Invite shared decision making and explain the healthcare provider's role in the decision making
"Recommendations"	• Explain healthcare provider recommendations • Explain possible risks and benefits of recommendations • Demonstrate respect with the recommendations of others to the health seeker
"Education"	• Assess the communication partners stage of change and readiness for change • Empower patients to use their own resources, strategies, and strengths toward health behavior change • Consider best practices when sharing information with communication partners (how much information do they already know, how much more do they want to know; provide information in chunks and monitor for their understanding, allow time for reflection of new information, and so on)
"Closure"	• Identify if there are any other issues to be shared in the encounter by the communication partner before ending the encounter • Ensure pace of the encounter is not rushed at its closing • Clarify follow-up steps for after the encounter is over and how the communication partner can be contacted (if necessary)
"With the team"	• Identify roles in the team • Share relevant information to members of the team to enhance collaboration • Cooperate with members of the team

Process (How Is Information Shared Among Communication Partners)

Communication between people

The basis for the communication in clinical practice is the patient-centered clinical method. The seminal publications from 1986 describe the methods and contrast the approach to the style of the time that was disease-specific and centered around the goal of attaining a diagnosis, rather than addressing the needs of the patient.[5] Clinicians are expected to facilitate the interview, guiding the patient through the history to elicit information, but also to delve into the patient's deep concerns, expectations, and context. The series of articles incorporate practical applications, including the labeling of categories that would be essential to explore with the patient. These are addressing the fears of the patient, exploring the patient's ideas about what the patient thinks may be going on, assessing the level of functioning of the patient, and how the illness may be impacting the patient's functioning, and finally, asking the patient explicitly about his or her expectations for the visit. These categories are known as FIFE (fears, ideas, function, and expectation).[6] For example, a young woman presents to the family practice office with a complaint of abdominal pain. The PA may ask her about her concern, which may be the pain, or, if given the opportunity to say more, may be the underlying fear that she has colon cancer, as a young friend was recently diagnosed with the disease. The PA may explore the idea of abdominal pain with the patient and how she perceives this as a sign of a serious disease that is incurable, because her friend is now on chemotherapy. The encounter can just focus on the series of symptoms, such as the pain descriptors, weight loss, change in stool, and the like, but to be patient-centered, the encounter would also include a discussion of how the abdominal pain is affecting the patient's level of functioning. Is she still able to work? To sleep through the night? This also helps the PA understand the level of severity of the presenting complaint. And, finally, the PA may ask the patient upfront, her expectations for the visit. Does she want a colonoscopy? An ultrasound? Reassurance? Understanding the expectations of the patient allows the clinician to better negotiate a management plan. In this case, for example, if the history supported a likely benign presentation of mild irritable bowel syndrome, further investigations may not be warranted, and some simple symptom management techniques may be suggested. However, if the presentation contained any red flags, further investigation may be warranted. The likelihood of the patient "buying in" to either management plan will very much depend on how it is presented. Being denied invasive investigations when one is expecting it will be hard to accept, if the conversation did not allow for the exploration of fears and expectations and the clinician explaining the rationale.

Common ground

The same investigators of the seminal work published outcomes on their training methods to family physicians. The perception of patients feeling they reached common ground with their provider, the use of fewer diagnostic tests, and improved health status (patient perceived wellness, and recovery from his or her presenting concern) all improved.[4] A more recent Cochrane review of the topic supports some of their findings, and some mixed conclusions, given the complexity of the topic and ability to "prove" its effect.[7]

This aspect of the patient-centered clinical method became popular and the acronym FIFE became a verb, as students may be encouraged to "FIFE" the patient during clinical skills simulation practice. "FIFE-ing" can become a checklist, and the mnemonic, for students and novice clinicians, has a tendency to be used in a formulaic manner. The exploration of the patient's context as related to his or her fears, ideas, and expectations requires genuine empathy. The use of empathy as a communication skill, however, requires an understanding of its purpose and role in the patient-centered clinical method to be genuine and effective. If the patient in our example states, "my friend is now on chemotherapy and I am worried," the response with the phrase "that must be very hard for you" can be otherwise (facetiously) stated "insert empathic phrase here." Consider an alternate response to the patient's fears with genuine empathy for her overall condition with the use of acknowledgment, reflection, and sometimes, prolonged silence. A response such as, "that sounds like you are really worried about your friend," followed by a pause and allowing time for the patient to say more, is a way to demonstrate empathy and allow the patient to share his or her illness experience in a genuine way that may help achieve common ground and alleviate suffering.

In a recent analysis of clinical encounters in primary and specialty care practices, it was noted that the clinician interrupts patients at about 11 seconds into the conversation when trying to elicit the patient's concerns. The patient's agenda was seldom sought, although more often (49% of encounters reviewed) in primary care settings than in specialty settings (20% of encounters reviewed). The investigators' message is, "Failure to elicit the patient's agenda reduces the chance that clinicians will orient the priorities of a clinical encounter toward specific aspects that matter to each patient."[8] As the PA is the front-line clinician, practicing effective communication strategies to illicit patient concerns will result in better care.

Trust

If an opera singer was told to go into a room, practice singing the aria in private, with no one else listening, and then told to come out of the room, and report on how it went, we would all question this approach. However, in the traditional education for the practice of medicine, that is what we did. Go see the patient, take a history, and report back on your findings. In modern, competency-based medical education, there is a push toward direct observation, whether in simulation or with real patients, to directly observe the competence of the learner. However, once out in practice, there is an assumption that the information gathered, physical examination maneuvers, and counseling and management plan are all in keeping with what the supervisor would consider competent. How is this achieved? Through trust.

As the practicing PA, there is an assumption that you have the communication skills necessary to conduct a thorough history. No one should have to check that the story you are reporting is correct. There is a trust that what the patient told you is what you are now documenting in the medical record, and, where applicable, reporting directly to your supervising physician.

How is that trust achieved? The answer is part of a larger issue of human nature and how trust is earned and reinforced. However, the simple answer, for the purposes of our discussion, is that if a PA has excellent communication skills, there is an assumption that his or her ability to assess the patient will be accurate and reliable. The PA and supervising physician have a symbiotic relationship. They rely on each other to provide the best patient care as their shared goal.

Cultural competence

Canada's multicultural society is considered a melting pot, and new Canadians are able to maintain their cultural or ethnic identities of origin. Freedom of religion and separation of church and state are cornerstones of our society. Culturally sensitive and culturally appropriate healthcare is an expectation of patients. More recently, physicians have spoken out about being harassed or mistreated by patients because of their own ethno-religious identities.[9] Addressing cultural competence in PA education has been written about elsewhere.[10,11] Simply reporting on the race of a patient, as has been studied in internal medicine, can lead to erroneous assumptions.[12] Along with considering the patient's context, being aware of the role of culture in the patient experience is paramount.

The "Process Skills" of communication are listed in **Table 3** with six subdomains and relevant learning outcomes.

Table 3	
Process skills of communication: subdomains and selected learning outcomes	
Process Skills[3] of Communication: Subdomains	**Examples of Learning Outcomes[3] in This Domain (As a Practicing PA, I Can...)**
"Characteristics of communication"	• Demonstrate confidence • Communicate with honesty • Demonstrate flexibility and adapt communication accordingly • Allow others time to reply and complete their thoughts (do not interrupt unless necessary to redirect) • Reflect back what you have heard
"Relationships and communication"	• Demonstrate willingness to work with people in different contexts (including cross-cultural communication) • Use inclusive language • Describe the perspectives of others on your team
"Emotions and communication"	• Demonstrate empathy (acknowledge the feelings, vulnerabilities, difficulties of others; avoid judgments and platitudes, validate the expression of others) • Monitor the emotional state of the communication partner and react accordingly • Recognize conflicts • Navigate through difficult conversations
"Verbal behavior"	• Set the agenda for the healthcare interaction • Prepare for the interaction (review available information, acknowledge available sources of information, anticipate potential challenges that may arise in the interaction) • Speak at an appropriate pace, tone, and volume • Use single questions • Use open-ended and closed-ended questions appropriately • Use verbal cues (reflect what was heard, use encouraging words, acknowledge what was said, paraphrase, minimally interrupt)
"Nonverbal behavior"	• Use appropriate eye contact • Use appropriate facial expressions and body language • Use nonverbal cues to support active listening (head nodding, pausing, undivided attention, not rushing)
"Communication modes"	• Demonstrate focus when in conversation (not being distracted by reading, writing, or typing) • Summarize encounters for medical records • Demonstrate organization • Provides resources when appropriate • Uses professional words and language and avoids jargon • Recognizes limitations of others • Advocates for others • Uses technologies appropriately

Perception (Reflecting On One's Own Position in the Context of a Communication Encounter)

The final domain of "perception" is more about internal realizations and growth than external impact. However, it is a testament to the complexity of the role of communicator. One needs the background knowledge (*why*), the content skill (*what*), and the process (*how*) to bring it all together. To be effective, PAs also need to reflect on their own abilities and impact that their communication has on others. This is the perception domain. One needs the knowledge to gain the skill to deliver the *how*. Yet, to continually improve, one needs to be self-aware and reflect on his or her own performance.

Developing a communication style may take some time and experience and requires insight into one's own behaviors. Practically, a PA may start by identifying his or her own emotional reactions in specific communication encounters. If one of the communication partners is becoming defensive, that emotion, often a threatening one, may easily transfer to the other partner in communication. Recognizing these emotions may not only be helpful to avoid escalating conflict but may also serve to promote wellness and avoid professional burnout.

Reflection remains one of the hardest skills to measure or evaluate. Reflection is a skill to be taught and honed and often does not come automatically to some. Separating one's objective performance (ie, *did I get all the relevant details of the patient's history?*) from the emotions of encounter (ie, *did my disapproval of this patient's behavior come across to the extent that the patient will refuse to take my advice?*) can be challenging for many, especially in difficult circumstances. Acknowledging these challenges is how we get better. PAs work in teams and with supervision, thus the opportunity for feedback from others should be accessible and valued. Feedback has been described as a "gift," wrapped up with a large bow (Cudmore J, personal communication, Toronto, Ontario, Canada, 2010). For the receiver, it is his or her choice to unwrap the gift, examine it closely, appreciate the thoughtful intent and inherent value, and decide how and where to best use the gift moving forward. Alternatively, the receiver of this "gift" of feedback may simply put it on a shelf, wrapped up and forgotten, or even put it in the trash. It is difficult to see oneself as others see us, and even harder still, to critique ourselves. As such, feedback becomes one of the most valuable gifts to cherish.

Table 4 lists three subdomains associated with the "Perceptual Skills" of communication. Examples of associated learning outcomes are included.

Table 4 Perceptual skills of communication: subdomains and selected learning outcomes	
Perceptual Skills[3] of Communication: Subdomains	Examples of Learning Outcomes[3] in This Domain (*As a Practicing PA, I Can…*)
"Impact of self"	• Recognize one's own personal context and emotion and how these impact one's own communication • Recognize trigger situations and one's personal response in these challenging encounters • Reflect on one's own emotional reactions • Demonstrate self-disclosure in appropriate context
"Self-evaluation"	• Describe the importance of reflection on practice • Identify the importance of ongoing professional development of one's communication skills • Reflect on communication encounters, identifying both strengths and areas for improvement
"External evaluation"	• Seek feedback from others on communication encounters • Use the feedback to help adjust or change future communication encounters

SUMMARY

Although the intrinsic skill of communication is a complex one, it remains a practical exercise to reduce the topic into a series of simplified parts, for the purposes of education and ongoing professional development. However, one cannot simply look at the role of communicator in healthcare as a series of finite learning outcomes or measurable tasks. Doing so may lessen the authenticity of the provider, especially when trying to emulate a task within the larger role of communicator.[13] Being able to document a succinct and comprehensive medical note after an encounter does not automatically mean that the patient felt that the verbal communication was effective or that their needs were met. Without having all the tools in the toolbox, using just one tool in isolation may seem indifferent or illegitimate. However, the caution remains to ensure the overall competence is not lost while teaching, learning, and demonstrating this complex ability.

When considering communication skills for PAs, the framework of using knowledge, exploring content, following process, and heightening perceptions can help both practicing PAs and other members of the healthcare team to break down the sometimes-esoteric topic into manageable domains and subdomains.

REFERENCES

1. Canadian Association of Physician Assistants. 2015. Available at: capa-acam.ca; https://capa-acam.ca/wp-content/uploads/2015/11/CanMEDS-PA.pdf. Accessed May 16, 2019.
2. Higgs J, McAllister L, Sefton A. Communication in the health sciences. 3rd edition. South Melbourne (Australia): Oxford University Press; 2012.
3. Denniston C, Molloy E, Nestel D, et al. Learning outcomes for communication skills across the health professions: a systematic literature review and qualitative synthesis. BMJ Open 2017;7:e014570.
4. Stewart M, Brown JB, Donner A, et al. The impact of patient-centered care on outcomes. J Fam Pract 2000;49(9):796–804.
5. Levenstein JH, McCracken EC, McWhinney IR. The patient-centred clinical method. 1. A model for the doctor-patient interaction in family medicine. Fam Pract 1986;3(1):24–30.
6. Brown J, Stewart M, McCracken E, et al. The patient-centred clinical method. 2. Definition and application. Fam Pract 1986;3(2):75–9.
7. Dwamena F, Holmes-Rovner M, Gaulden CM, et al. Interventions for providers to promote a patient-centred approach in clinical consultations. Cochrane Database Syst Rev 2012;(12):CD003267.
8. Singh Ospina N, Phillips KA, Rodriguez-Gutierrez R, et al. Eliciting the patient's agenda- secondary analysis of recorded clinical encounters. J Gen Intern Med 2019;34(1):36–40.
9. Chattopadhyay P, Goldhar K. What can doctors do when they face racism from the people they're trying to help? The Current (Canada): CBC Radio; 2019.
10. Kelly P. Should we rethink how we teach cultural competency in physician assistant education? J Physician Assist Educ 2012;23(3):42–5.
11. LeLacheur S, Straker H. Culture, diversity, race, and the standards: assessing and addressing the hidden curricula. J Physician Assist Educ 2011;22(2):34–7.
12. Acquaviva KD, Mintz M. Perspective: are we teaching racial profiling? The dangers of subjective determinations of race and ethnicity in case presentations. Acad Med 2010;85(4):702–5.
13. Salmon P, Young B. Creativity in clinical communication: from communication skills to skilled communication. Med Education 2011;45:217–26.

Collaboration for Physician Assistants: Working as a Team

Sylvia Langlois, BHSc, MSc, OT Reg (ON)[a,b,*],
Dean Lising, PT, BSc, BscPT, MHSc[a,c]

KEYWORDS

- Team-based healthcare • Interprofessional teams
- Interprofessional communication • Team process

KEY POINTS

- Interprofessional competencies guide team-based healthcare to provide optimal patient-centered care and address the quadruple aim outlined by the Institute for Healthcare Improvement.
- Team assessments provide an opportunity to consider how a team is functioning. Follow-up with a debrief and team reflection enables enhanced team process.
- A commitment to respectful interactions among team members establishes psychological safety for the team, which in turn enhances team communication and collaboration.
- Interprofessional communication enables teamwork. Strategies to facilitate communication among team members and approaches to managing conflict scenarios provide foundational instruction to enhancing team process.

INTRODUCTION

Concerns about increasing complexity of patients' health conditions and comorbidities, errors that occur in the process of care delivery, and rising costs have necessitated an examination of traditional practices in healthcare delivery models. Over the past two decades, healthcare services have evolved from uniprofessional (activities specific to one profession) and multiprofessional interactions (healthcare

Disclosure Statement: The authors have nothing to disclose.
[a] Centre for Interprofessional Education, University of Toronto, University Health Network, Toronto Western Hospital, 399 Bathurst St., Nassau Annex (Entrance), Toronto, ON M5T 2S8, Canada; [b] Department of Occupational Science and Occupational Therapy, Faculty of Medicine, University of Toronto, Toronto, Ontario, Canada; [c] Department of Physical Therapy, Faculty of Medicine, University of Toronto, 160 – 500 University Avenue, Toronto, ON M5G 1V7, Canada
* Corresponding author. Centre for Interprofessional Education, University of Toronto University Health Network, Toronto Western Hospital, 399 Bathurst Street. Nassau Annex (Entrance), Toronto, ON M5T 2S8, Canada.
E-mail address: s.langlois@utoronto.ca

Physician Assist Clin 5 (2020) 61–77
https://doi.org/10.1016/j.cpha.2019.08.007
2405-7991/20/© 2019 Elsevier Inc. All rights reserved.
physicianassistant.theclinics.com

professions engaging in patient care in a parallel approach) to an enhanced focus on interprofessional, team-based care models. Team-based healthcare is defined as

> ...the provision of health services to individuals, families, and/or their communities by at least two health providers who work collaboratively with patients and their caregivers—to the extent preferred by each patient—to accomplish shared goals within and across settings to achieve coordinated, high-quality care.[1]

Team-based care can be challenging given the complexity of professions, roles, settings across different sectors, and varying practices. Questions arise as to the nature of teams, the types of communication and collaboration that best support interprofessional team-based care, and strategies that enable growing partnerships with patients and family members.

Although team-based healthcare is recognized as optimal practice, what is needed are approaches to promote not only teamwork but also high-functioning teams. In support of this goal, the Interprofessional Education Collaborative (IPEC) has created a framework[2] to address interprofessional competencies needed in practice environments. Although there are four competencies outlined in the framework, this article focuses primarily on two in order to deepen understanding of teams and interprofessional communication strategies that are relevant to the practice of physician assistants (PAs). The discussion begins with an anchor in the relationship-centered care framework.

RELATIONSHIP-CENTERED CARE

PA relationships in teams are key to interprofessional collaborative practice and can be understood within the framework for relationship-centered care.[3,4] There are four key interconnected, relational dimensions to this framework:

1. Practitioner to patient: patients are the center of healthcare practice and practitioners are responsive to their needs in a shared decision-making process.[5,6]
2. Practitioner to practitioner: at the core of collaborative practice is the relationship between and among practitioners where collaborative conversations and diversity are valued to work toward shared understanding.
3. Practitioner to self: this dimension addresses self-awareness and reflective practice with recognition of one's own perspectives, values, and biases on potential impact on key stakeholders.
4. Practitioner to community: this dimension emphasizes that relationships occur in community contexts, which play an important role in the health and well-being of individuals, inclusive of communities of patients, and communities where patients live.

INTERPROFESSIONAL COMPETENCIES

Interprofessional education and practice in the United States are guided by the competencies outlined by IPEC. In healthcare, competencies are described as "Integrated enactment of knowledge, skills, values, and attitudes that define working together across the professions, with other healthcare workers, and with patients, along with families and communities, as appropriate to improve health outcomes in specific care contexts."[2] These competencies are designed to address the quadruple aim,[7,8] an approach widely adopted to optimize the performance of the health system.[9] These specific aims are to

- Improve the patient experience of care
- Improve the health of populations
- Reduce the per capita cost of healthcare
- Improve the work life of healthcare providers, clinicians, and staff

The IPEC framework (**Fig. 1**) depicts the relationship of the four competency domains. Two domains, values and ethics for interprofessional practice and roles and responsibilities for collaborative practice, are summarized. The remaining two are discussed more fully.

VALUES AND ETHICS FOR INTERPROFESSIONAL PRACTICE

Values and ethics are foundational to collaborative practice. Attitudes and thoughts drive behaviors; thus, a commitment to honoring the relationships (patients, family members, and team members) implicit in healthcare delivery is critical. Specific IPEC subcompetencies in this construct address:

- Centering interprofessional healthcare on the interests of patients and populations
- Embracing cultural diversity of patients and team members

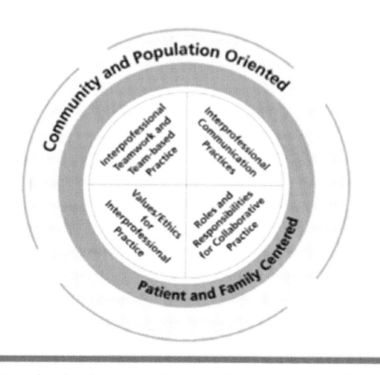

Fig. 1. Interprofessional collaboration competency domain. (Interprofessional Education Collaborative. (2016). Core competencies for interprofessional collaborative practice: 2016 update. Washington, DC: Interprofessional Education Collaborative. Available at: https://nebula.wsimg.com/2f68a39520b03336b41038c370497473?AccessKeyId=DC06780E69ED19E2B3A5&disposition=0&alloworigin=1.)

- Respecting values, roles, and expertise of other healthcare team members
- Collaborating with patients and team members
- Developing relationships based on trust
- Demonstrating ethical conduct and quality in care management
- Demonstrating honest and integrity in relationships

In their realist synthesis, Hewitt and colleagues[10] identified important mechanisms contributing to interprofessional teamwork. Those relevant to the described foundational values and ethics include a shared sense of purpose (common values and vision enhancing consistency in care and commitment to the work), support, and value (team members support each other and feel their work is valued by others; they demonstrate trust and respect).

Roles and Responsibilities for Collaborative Practice

Understanding the roles and responsibilities of other healthcare team members is critical to the function of a team that has a holistic, patient-centered approach. Some of the subcompetencies outlined include

- Recognizing one's own limits
- Communicating the team approach, including roles and responsibilities of the other healthcare professionals
- Integrating the scope of practice of other healthcare team members
- Communicating with team members to ensure responsibilities for components of the care plan are clarified

PAs can develop their understanding of roles and responsibilities of other healthcare professionals by learning about, from, and with other professional colleagues in opportunities, such as asking questions to clarify roles of other professions or formal collaborative education activities. With enhanced role understanding, PAs are empowered to respond to expressed and/or observed patient needs.

The discussion of the remaining two competencies, interprofessional teamwork and team-based practice and interprofessional communication practices, begins with a review of some of the barriers to collaborative practice. Although interprofessional teamwork is recognized as an optimal approach, PAs and other team members acknowledge that the ideal is not always achieved. Healthcare delivery spans both hospital and community settings, each with its own concomitant complexities and challenges to collaboration. Additionally, communication between hospitals and community-based healthcare services can result in inefficiencies and ineffective processes. Healthcare providers, however, can use measures to overcome system limitations to be successful in the provision of excellent care. Awareness of the barriers and an understanding of contributing factors support clinician ability to work beyond the system limitations. A review of the literature identifies some of the contextual, organizational, and team challenges to communication and collaborative practice that span the described competencies as

- Spatial and temporal organization of working space that can limit communication among team members[11]
- Poor management with inefficiencies in scheduling or staffing, limiting time or opportunities to work together[12]
- Patriarchy or gender norms that can affect communication[13]
- Perceived or actual power of professional groups that can have an impact on the creation of a safe environment for communication[13]

- Hierarchy of professions or roles that can affect patient care due to discomfort in communicating and sharing important information[12,13]
- Poor training to address nontechnical competencies related to communication and collaboration[13]
- Poor communication among team members, including inaccurate interpretation and timeliness of messages[12]
- Interpersonal and interprofessional conflict[12]
- Perceived or actual lack of competence of team members[12]
- Inadequate understanding of healthcare provider roles.[12]

Shared decision making and goal setting are foundational components of patient-centered, team-based care; however, some team member behaviors can impede this important collaborative function. Prystajeckya and colleagues[14] reported that the following activities impaired achievement of team-based patient goals:

- Variable team member attendance at meetings
- Exchanges of information that are not relevant to monitoring or setting of goals
- Inconsistent team member contributions
- Shifting team leadership patterns

INTERPROFESSIONAL TEAMS AND TEAMWORK

Recognizing that PAs are increasingly integrated in teams, consideration of team process and role in influencing team dynamics is critical to navigate the previously discussed contextual, organizational, and team challenges. The IPEC framework identifies competencies in the domain of team and teamwork as applying relationship-building values and the principles of team dynamics to perform effectively in different team roles to optimize safe, quality care and population health.[2] In order to apply this competency to team-based care, reflective questions related to teamwork need to be considered and key team practices applied that can support their collaborative work and relationship-centered care to achieve high team performance and optimal patient outcomes.

What Is a Team?

A team is defined as a group of people with complementary skills who are committed to a common purpose, performance goals, and approach for which they hold themselves mutually accountable.[15] The World Health Organization expands on the concept of team-based care to be inclusive of both clinical and nonclinical health-related work, such as diagnosis, treatment, surveillance, health communications, management, and sanitation engineering, key roles sometimes missed when considering team processes.[16] Teams are encouraged to reflect on and challenge their traditional notion of a team, considering members who have both a regular and/or intermittent presence. The concept of team should also include providers, leaders, and patient/client/family or learner representatives who are part of the patient journey, including involvement of interorganizational or intersectoral roles.

Why Is Team Process Important?

Team processes are defined as a group-level phenomenon that has an impact on clinical tasks, quality of care, and safety and refers to dynamics, such as communication, collaboration, coordination, conflict, leadership, and

---

Consider this scenario through a PA PERSPECTIVE:

You are walking along the corridor of an operating theater suite when you hear a call for help. You respond automatically and enter an anesthetic room to find an anesthetist and an operating department practitioner trying to intubate an already cyanosed patient. Glancing up at the monitors, you observe that the patient's oxygen saturation is falling. You know the anesthetist and the operating department practitioner; they are experienced and diligent and you respect them. Another anesthetist arrives to help and a fellow nursing colleague walks in behind you, carrying a tracheostomy tray, but no one seems to notice the other nurse. She puts the tray on the side, next to the mini-tracheostomy kit. The surgeon walks in and appears aloof and dismissive of nursing staff, which you find intimidating and puts you on edge. This is now a busy room with six people, and the consultants continue in their efforts to try to intubate the patient, with little success. The patient is motionless and anesthetized but receiving no oxygen and you know instinctively this is an emergency. It is not at all clear who is in charge and you do not understand why the consultants are not trying other ways to secure the patient's airway to provide much-needed oxygen. You leave the room and phone the intensive care unit (ICU), telling them of the emergency in the operating theater and of the patient's respiratory distress, and they immediately offer a bed. You return to the anesthetic room and announce: "A bed is available in ICU." The three consultants turn to you because no one has spoken as assertively or as loudly as you in the past few minutes. They look at you dismissively, in a way that seems to translate as, "What's wrong? You are over-reacting." You are surprised at their response and start to doubt if you have interpreted the situation correctly. It looks like surgical access is needed, the tracheostomy set is on the side, and you are wondering why are they not using it or even discussing it as an option. You begin to feel uncomfortable under their glare and again doubt your assessment of the situation—surely they know what they are doing. You walk out and cancel the ICU bed. You learn later that the patient's condition did not improve and she needed to go to ICU after all. You learn later still that the patient died.

Could things have been done differently? Could the team have responded more effectively?

---

decision making.[17] There is a growing focus on the importance of team's attention to their team process and dynamics to improve their effectiveness and reduce error. Strong team functioning has been shown to be related to improved patient outcomes, staff satisfaction, and less burnout.[17–19] In a narrative review of four reports of ethnographic studies of patient safety in UK hospitals, Dixon-Woods[20] highlighted interprofessional team dynamics and communication as key to patient safety challenges, with teams failing to share important information or coordinate activities influenced by professional boundaries and hierarchies.

The following case study[21] based on a true scenario illustrates the potential impact of team process on safety and medical error.[21]

This is based on the true story of Elaine Bromiley, who underwent elective corrective surgery and septoplasty; challenging team dynamics and ineffective communication between professionals led to the devastating tragic outcome of this scenario.[21] As in this example, a high-performing team member could still produce an inadequate result due to being part of a poorly performing team. Likewise, a team member, such as a PA, could perform less than optimally on a high-performing team that collectively produces a highly successful outcome.[22] Teams that assess, learn together, and debrief on key team processes have been shown to produce strong outcomes. A meta-analysis found that healthcare team training was linked to positive outcomes within the healthcare context, including reduced patient mortality, reduced medical error, and improved teamwork on-the-job.[23] This applies not only to teams collaborating for care but also to teams collaborating on quality-improvement and safety initiatives. Santana noted that successful quality=improvement and safety teams reframed interprofessional tensions, disagreement, and conflict and saw this as a necessary step in the redesign of a complex, interdisciplinary care process.[24]

How Can Team Processes Be Optimized?

Given the complexity of teamwork and team processes, there is no one tool or practice that resolves all team challenges. It is important for PAs, in collaboration with other team members, however, to consider some key team processes, such as optimizing psychological safety, team norming, assessment, and debriefing, that may support a team, improve outcomes, and minimize error.

How to Optimize Psychological Safety?

Edmondson[25] defines psychological safety as a shared belief among members that the team is a safe place for interpersonal risk taking. Psychological safety is supported through encouraging respectful interactions and consistently addressing disrespectful behavior. Creating a team climate where raising a dissenting view is expected and respected, error reporting is welcomed, and where team members are open to offer ideas, questions, and concerns is important.[25] A scoping review examining team dynamics involved in quality-improvement initiatives reviewed literature on psychosocial traits and noted successful leadership in the presence of hierarchical differences may be dependent on a particularly inclusive leadership style.[26] Nembhard and Edmondson[27] identified the link between displays of leader inclusiveness and the teams' reports of psychological safety. Interestingly, there was an increase in overall psychological safety when individuals who were perceived to have higher status intentionally invited perspectives from other members. Considering the key roles of PAs as leaders and team members, encouraging a climate of psychological safety for themselves and their colleagues can produce safer and higher-quality care. Furthermore, psychological safety can be developed, supported, and enhanced through team development and reflection activities that engage members and leaders to consider the team climate and their role in supporting it. This is particularly successful if leaders, both formal and informal, role model and encourage psychological safety as a key team and organizational norm.

How Can Team Norms Support Successful Interaction?

Norms are the traditions, behavioral standards, and unwritten rules that govern how professionals function when gathered and can be unspoken or openly acknowledged. In order to practice collaboratively, healthcare team members should agree on team processes, rules, and practices for the team and service users.[28] These norms may be implicit and unspoken, but the literature supports the value of naming and explicitly co-creating these norms together. Organizational norms related to shared decision making and stability in team membership were identified as important to developing psychological safety in interprofessional teams.[29] Positive norms and understanding of team rules have been shown to achieve clinical goals, delineate professional boundaries, improve staff morale, enhance support between team members, and facilitate conflict resolution and problem solving[30–33] (**Box 1**).

How Can Team Function Be Assessed?

Formalized team assessments facilitate team-based reflections on process. Given the growing number of surveys, questionnaires, and learner or team assessment instruments reported in the literature, teams should scrutinize tools to ensure they

---

Box 1
Example of co-created team norms (Centre for Interprofessional Education, University of Toronto)

Here is a sampling of team norms utilized by an interprofessional education and practice team as a starting point for other teams to consider in co-creation of their own norms. These team norms are the foundation for shared work, interactions, and meetings. They are displayed in the team meeting room and referred to regularly in team meetings and debriefings.

- We will communicate with honesty and respect.
- We will have regular reflection as a team.
- We will share leadership, so others can learn and grow.
- We will ensure a safe environment where ideas can be shared.
- We will celebrate our successes and each other.
- We will give and receive feedback freely.
- We will hold each other accountable to our commitments.

---

choose one that fits their context. Purpose of the tool, intended population, usability, cost/training factors, psychometrics, and analysis should all be considered in the selection process. One example of a comprehensive team assessments is the Assessment of Interprofessional Team Collaboration Scale (AITCS),[34] which can provide valuable information on multiple elements of team-based care and competencies. There are also often shorter modified versions of comprehensive team assessment tools with fewer items (eg, modified AITCS[35] and Team Climate Inventory[36]), which may be easier for busy teams to complete. There are also scales to measure psychological safety of a team and the level of risk-taking on a team.[25] Hospital teams and leadership in the Toronto Academic Health Science Network, Toronto, utilized a combination of these comprehensive team assessment tools to support team competency education, action planning, and reflection on team climate, and psychological safety. Team assessment combined with reflection can enable PAs, in collaboration with other team members and leaders, to better understand their climate and support goals, and plan improvement initiatives to enhance their practice.

How Do Reflection and Debriefing Foster Team Dynamics?

The Elaine Bromiley case is one of many examples where, in the aftermath of an incident or a near-miss, a team can debrief and reflect together to prevent future error. Critical incident analysis involves focusing on an event, including analyzing the circumstances surrounding it, the actions of those involved, responses to the event, and the outcomes to understand how practice can be improved.[37] Teams need not be limited by critical incident debriefing; debriefing and reflective activities can be added to routine practices, collaborative learning situations, and simulations.[38] A debriefing to reflect on what went well and where improvements may be possible can occur after regular team interactions. One meta-analysis of 46 studies found that debriefings improved individual and team performance relative to a control group by approximately 25%.[39] Reyes and colleagues[40] developed best practice guidelines and a useful, easy-to-implement debrief tool outline. This tool takes as little as 10 minutes at the end of a meeting and can facilitate a debriefing reflection, and action planning (**Box 2**).

As a healthcare provider, I am acutely aware of the quality of services provided and the nature of interactions among professionals. My 90-year old mother who lives in the community with minimal support became ill when she contracted influenza, leading to an exacerbation of chronic obstructive lung disease that progressed to double pneumonia and a subsequent collapsed left lung. We took her to an emergency department when her breathing became labored. While waiting for a bed in emergency, her condition deteriorated rapidly. She was admitted to an ICU bed for five days and then to a ward bed for recovery. Because of the intense need for beds during the influenza outbreak, the team was prepared to discharge her within two days of admission to the ward. At that point, she had only been up for very brief walks in her room. The discharge was planned without consideration of the level of function required to live in a community setting. No one had checked basic self-care skills or assessed her ability to manage meal preparation or household tasks. I raised my concern for the apparent lack of coordination with the senior resident.

While we were discussing the situation in the hallway, the resident suggested we have the conversation *with* my mother. Within five minutes, she had gathered the discharge planner, social worker, nurse, physiotherapist, and occupational therapist to stand around my mother's bed. Together we talked about what was needed at home and collaboratively created a plan of community and home care support to ensure she would be safe on discharge. She was discharged and continued to recover at home with support from nursing (to manage the incision from the collapsed lung and monitor health), physiotherapy (to improve ambulation and balance after extended bedrest), occupational therapy (to determine supports and modifications needed to manage daily activities), social work (to teach her to manage the anxiety that had resulted from a traumatic medical procedure when her lung collapsed) and a personal support worker. Without this degree of team communication and collaboration that included my and my mother's input, both in hospital and in the community, her discharge would not likely have been successful.

Box 2
Quick team debriefing outline

1. Set the stage (30–60 seconds)
   - Explain why you are conducting a debriefing and what the team will be discussing.
   - "This is a quick opportunity to learn from our experience. Let's look at how we handled this [situation, project, event, meeting, shift]: what we did well or could improve."
   - "Let's consider how we worked as a team, in addition to any technical issues."
   - If there are any boundaries or non-negotiables, let the team know what is off limits.

2. Ask the team for their observations (5–20 minutes)
   - What happened?
   - What did we do well? What challenges did we face?
   - What should we do differently or focus on next time?
   - What could help us be more effective? Anything we need?

3. Add your observations/recommendations and confirm understanding (5–10 minutes)
   - Reinforce their observations, or if you noticed something different, share your view of what happened or needs to happen in the future.
   - Be sure any feedback you provide is clear, actionable, and focuses on the work, not personal traits.

4. Summarize any agreed-on actions or focus for the future (5 minutes)
   - Be clear about who will do what, when…and how this will help the team.
   - Specify when and how you will follow-up to assess progress (eg, next debriefing).

Tip: ask the team for their perceptions first. Then if possible, acknowledge one thing that you could have done differently or that you will focus on in the future. This will make it easier for team members to voice their own observations or concerns.

Tip: If the team does not discuss teamwork, ask, "How well did we work together as a team?"

Perhaps ask 1 or 2 specific questions, such as:

HOW WELL DID WE...
+ Communicate/share info
+ Monitor/provide backup
+ Coordinate with "outsiders"
+ Speak up/challenge one another
+ Ask for/offer help
+ Handle conflict
+ Share/allocate resources
+ Prepare/plan

HOW CLEAR WERE OUR...
+ Roles/assignments
+ Goals/priorities

Basic assumption of team debriefing: "We're all competent and well-intentioned people who want to do our best. This is about getting better at what we do."

Adapted from www.gOEbase.com.

INTERPROFESSIONAL COMMUNICATION PRACTICES

Communication and teamwork are inextricably linked; effective communication enables teamwork and optimal patient care. Communication can occur in both formal and informal formats. Essential formalized team communication usually takes the form of ward rounds or family meetings. Yet, equally essential to patient care are informal meetings that occur among different team members or the patient/client or family. These meetings may be chance encounters or impromptu and are recognized as enhancing a holistic understanding of a patient's needs and goals of care. An example of the value of such encounters is described in the following anecdote.

STRATEGIES TO ENHANCE TEAMWORK AND TEAM COMMUNICATION

Effective communication influences the healthcare team dynamic and enhances the quality of the work environment but, more critically, has an impact on the delivery of safe, optimal patient care. The Joint Commission on Accreditation of Healthcare Organizations, in an analysis of more than 2000 critical incidents, reported that more than 70% were linked to poor interprofessional communication (Leonard and colleagues[41]). Recognizing that communication ultimately leads to better patient outcomes, teams can consider a selection of tools and programs that serve to facilitate the communication process to address patient-centeredness and safety. Two potential approaches frequently in the healthcare literature are described:

1. Team development and communication programs: team education and skill training, such as Team Strategies and Tools to Enhance Performance and Patient Safety (TeamSTEPPS): can enhance teamwork and optimize high quality, safe patient care. This evidence-based program, originally developed by the Department of Defense and the Agency for Healthcare Research and Quality, has been implemented widely.[42] Core dimensions include team structure, leadership, situation monitoring, mutual support, and communication. The TeamSTEPPS program has been widely cited as an approach in various clinical

settings, including outpatient clinics,[43] operating rooms,[44] obstetrics and neonatal ICUs,[45] long-term care,[46] and emergency departments.[47] Although improvement in communication and patient safety after completion of the program is described, there are concerns that the newly acquired teamwork behaviors are not sustained over time. Studies have demonstrated that the process of change is incremental and that it takes time[48]; yet, conversely, a decline in both attitudes and knowledge retention one year after completion of the program has been reported.[49] To sustain desired behaviors and attitudes, ongoing training is recommended.[49,50]

2. Communication tools: situation-background-assessment-recommendation (SBAR) is a communication tool that was originally designed for the military; it provides a concise approach to communication among team members.[51] The SBAR system can be used for patient reports, shift changes, handoffs, and unit transfers. Communication involves following these four steps:

   a. Situation—this description of the situation should be brief and succinct, identifying the patient, the problem, severity, and a brief history.
   b. Background—the background includes relevant history and test results and any information to further support the clinical situation addressed.
   c. Assessment—this step includes the clinician's assessment of the perceived situation, including what might be happening, potential mechanisms involved, assessment of severity, and consideration of the options.
   d. Recommendation—at this point, recommended actions or suggestions are stated.

This communication strategy is often used by nurses and physicians but can also include other healthcare professionals in interprofessional contexts.[50,52,53] The Joint Commission and the Institute for Healthcare Improvement have recommended the use of SBAR as best practice to enhance teamwork and foster patient safety.[54]

As described previously, effective communication strategies sit at the core of successful team-based collaboration. Anyone working in team environments, however, is aware of the potential conflicts that can occur among health professionals. Little is written regarding conflict experiences specific to PAs; yet, as part of the healthcare team, their experiences with challenging interactions with colleagues are inevitable, just as they are for other team members. Although deemed inevitable, most choose to avoid rather than directly deal with conflict; however, the use of appropriate conflict management competencies can be constructive, thereby enhancing decision making and outcomes. Various strategies for managing conflict among team members have been recommended. In one example, *Crucial Conversations*,[55] investigators describe the following steps to manage conversations in conflict situations:

1. Start with heart: identify what is at stake. Determine the importance of the conversation.
2. Learn to look: attempt to identify a mutual purpose. Reflect on the conversation, determining if dialogue or defensiveness is evident, making an effort to focus on the former.
3. Make it safe: attempt to create a comfortable, safe environment when conversations stray from dialogue.
4. Master your story: identify the facts behind the story.
5. State your path: state the facts from one's own perspective in such a way that other(s) can share their perspectives in a safe environment.
6. Explore others' path: ask questions and explore the perspective of the other person. With enhanced understanding, consider where there is agreement and where there are differences.

7. Move to action: work toward a consensus regarding next steps, documenting the arrangement.

Similar steps are described in other conflict management approaches. At the core is a commitment to address issues and demonstrate leadership to achieve the needed resolution. PAs, like other team members, are positioned to lead the process, supported by excellent tools and approaches.

Earlier in this article, the barriers to collaborative practice are identified. Following the discussion of teams and team functioning, facilitators and enablers to collaborative practice should be considered as described in the literature.

- Nonhierarchical workplace structures and communication patterns[56,57]
- Shared leadership approaches to enable collaboration[56]
- Commitment to collaboration[56]
- Mutual respect and trust[56,58]
- Commitment to working collaboratively[56]
- Protocols that enable collaboration[56]
- Team-focused rather than profession-focused goals[57]
- Regular communication (formal and informal) among team members[11,56,58]
- Appreciation of roles in healthcare that lead to holistic response to patient needs[11]
- Approachability of healthcare providers[11]
- Collaborative goal setting, involving appropriate team members and the patient and/or family members[58]
- Mutual accountability and acknowledgment of interdependence of team member roles[58,59]
- A patient-partnered approach where competition for healthcare professional time with a patient is addressed[57]

FINAL REFLECTIONS ON TEAMS

The conceptualization of collaborative practice, as defined previously, is typically focused on healthcare team members who are colocated. Yet, even in bounded hospital environments, there is fluidity regarding the constitution of teams and which healthcare professionals perceive themselves as members of the team and at what points of care. In their editorial, Dow and colleagues[60] encouraged readers to expand the concept of interprofessional practice to include collaboration as it occurs in networks. Subsequently, Reeves and colleagues[61] argued that teams and team working should not be regarded as moving along a single, linear, hierarchical spectrum from weak to strong but rather as a more nuanced conceptualization, in which the team design is matched to clinical purpose(s) and patient needs. In summary, they described the categories of team arrangements ranging from interprofessional teamwork (inclusive of core team-based elements including, but not restricted to, shared team identity, clarity, interdependence, integration, and shared responsibility. Team tasks are regarded, in general, as unpredictable, urgent, and complex) to less integration and interdependence toward an interprofessional network (shared team identify, clarity of roles goals, interdependence, integration, and shared responsibility are not as important; tasks are viewed as more predictable, less complex, and less urgent).

As PAs, consider the type of interactions with both clinical and nonclinical team members and interprofessional work required in the context of various conceptualizations of teams and the impact on delivering patient-centered care. Some of the following considerations may be helpful if practice may be more in a networking arrangement:

1. Practice in a patient-centered manner when communicating virtually using a network approach. How are patient goals identified, communicated, and addressed when health professionals are not colocated? How are patients and family members included in the shared decision-making process?
2. Determine appropriate methods of communication that involve all appropriate health professionals and foster shared decision-making. How are conflicts or differing priorities communicated and resolved by all involved?
3. Determine and follow guidelines for timely interprofessional communication and appropriate follow-up so that tasks are not inadvertently neglected.
4. Identify appropriate mechanisms for referrals to other health professionals and or other agencies. How will information from these referrals be documented and communicated to all who need to be informed to make appropriate revisions to the care plan?
5. Define mechanisms for identifying and enacting leadership roles.

COLLABORATIVE LEADERSHIP

Previously the IPEC competency framework, 1 of 5 international competency frameworks (United Kingdom Australia, Japan, United States,and Canada), is described. Although there are many similarities among competencies or capabilities identified, one that is unique appears in the Canadian Interprofessional Health Collaborative framework,[62] with an additional focus in the collaborative leadership domain. It considers determination of who will engage in group leadership roles through collaborative decision making, depending on the demands of the situation or task. Specifically, collaborative leadership addresses how to advance interdependent relationships, facilitate decision making, and support co-creation of an environment that fosters shared leadership and collaborative practice.[62] Leadership occurs in a relational context; collaborative leadership seeks to strengthen relationships to create an environment where trust becomes the foundation of interactions. Collaborative communication moves organizational or team-based decision making beyond the silos of profession-specific interactions enabling attainment of goals.

PAs can enable collaborative leadership by considering the following questions:

- How can interdependence of relationships and decision-making process be understood in the context of their team and situation?
- Determine what type of leadership is needed for the context. What leadership strengths are needed?
- Who are the most appropriate people to lead?
- How can collaborative leadership be fostered/supported in the context?
- What can be done to create an environment of trust?

SUMMARY

PAs work in interprofessional teams where team performance and the practice of other professions are interdependent. Attention to team process and team development has been shown to produce positive team and patient outcomes. Individuals and teams often focus more attention, however, on clinical skill development than interprofessional teamwork and communication practices. Explicit focus on key elements, such as team psychological safety, norming, communication, debriefing, and team assessment, can enhance the practice of PAs, improve quality of care, and reduce safety risks and errors. Additionally, reflection is important—reflection on how the team is defined, team process, and the context where the team practices, and recognizing the different types of interactions that exist in settings, such as primary care, community, and hospital teams. Given the changes in the healthcare system, increasing complexity of patient conditions, decreased financial and human resources, and changing scopes of practices and roles, PAs can be proactive in developing interprofessional competencies and positioning themselves for potential collaborative leadership roles. PAs are well located to support teamwork and influence the transformation of the healthcare system.

REFERENCES

1. Naylor MD, Coburn KD, Kurtzman ET, et al. Inter-professional team-based primary care for chronically ill adults: State of the science. Unpublished white paper presented at the ABIM Foundation meeting to Advance Team-Based Care for the Chronically Ill in Ambulatory Settings. Philadelphia, PA, March 24–25, 2010.
2. Interprofessional Education Collaborative. Core competencies for interprofessional collaborative practice: 2016 update. Washington, DC: Interprofessional Education Collaborative; 2016. Accessed June 14, 2019.
3. Pew-Fetzer Task Force on Advancing Psychosocial Health Education. Health professions education and relationship-centered care. San Francisco (CA): Pew Health Professions Commission; 1994.
4. Beach MC, Inui T, Relationship-Centered Care Research Network. Relationship-centered care: a constructive reframing. J Gen Intern Med 2006;21(Suppl 1):S3–8.
5. Hojat M, Vergare M, Maxwell K, et al. The devil is in the third year: a longitudinal study of erosion of empathy in medical school. Acad Med 2009;84(9):1182–91.
6. Neumann M, Edelhauser F, Tauschel D, et al. Empathy decline and its reasons: a systematic review of studies with medical students and residents. Acad Med 2011;86:996–1009.
7. Berwick DM, Nolan TW, Whittington J. The Triple Aim: care, health, and cost. Health Aff (Millwood) 2008;27(3):759–69.
8. Bodenheimer T, Sinsky C. From Triple to Quadruple Aim: care of the patient requires care of the provider. Ann Fam Med 2014;12(6):573–6.
9. Freeley D. Institute for healthcare improvement the triple aim or the quadruple aim? Four points to help set your strategy. 2017. Available at: http://www.ihi.org/communities/blogs/the-triple-aim-or-the-quadruple-aim-four-points-to-help-set-your-strategy. Accessed June 14, 2019.
10. Hewitt G, Sims S, Harris R. Using realist synthesis to understand the mechanisms of interprofessional teamwork in health and social care. J Interprof Care 2014;28(6):501–6.
11. Burm S, Boese K, Faden L, et al. Recognising the importance of informal communication events in improving collaborative care. BMJ Qual Saf 2019;28:289–95.
12. Soemantri D, Kambey DR, Yusra RY, et al. The supporting and inhibiting factors of interprofessional collaborative practice in a newly established teaching hospital. J Interprof Educ Pract 2019;15:149–56.
13. Jayasuriya-Illesinghe V, Guruge S, Gamage B, et al. Interprofessional work in operating rooms: a qualitative study from Sri Lanka. BMC Surg 2016;16:61.
14. Prystajecky M, Lee T, Abonyi S, et al. A case study of healthcare providers' goals during interprofessional rounds. J Interprof Care 2017;31(4):463–9.
15. Katzenbach JR, Smith DK. The wisdom of teams. New York: Harper Collins; 1994. p. 45.

16. World Health Organization. Framework for action on interprofessional education & collaborative practice. 2010. Available at: https://apps.who.int/iris/bitstream/handle/10665/70185/WHO_HRH_HPN_10.3_eng.pdf?sequence=1. Accessed June 14, 2019.
17. Lemieux-Charles L, McGuire WL. What do we know about healthcare team effectiveness? A review of the literature. Med Care Res Rev 2006;63:263–300.
18. Helfrich CD, Dolan ED, Simonetti J, et al. Elements of team-based care in a patient centered medical home are associated with lower burnout among VA primary care employees. J Gen Intern Med 2014;29(2):659–66.
19. Gittell JH, Fairfield KM, Bierbaum B, et al. Impact of relational coordination on quality of care, postoperative pain and functioning, and length of stay: a nine-hospital study of surgical patients. Med Care 2000;38(8):807–19.
20. Dixon-Woods M. Why is patient safety so hard? A selective review of ethnographic studies. J Health Serv Res Policy 2010;15(1):11–6.
21. Reid J, Bromiley M. Clinical human factors: the need to speak up and improve patient safety. Nurs Stand 2010;26(35):35–40.
22. Hodges BD, Lingard L. The question of competence: reconsidering medical education in the twenty-first century. Ithaca (NY): ILR Press; 2012.
23. Hughes AM, Gregory ME, Joseph DL. Saving lives: a meta-analysis of team training in healthcare. J Appl Psychol 2016;101(9):1266–304.
24. Santana C, Curry LA, Nembhard IM, et al. Behaviors of successful interdisciplinary hospital quality improvement teams. J Hosp Med 2011;6:501–6.
25. Edmondson AC. Psychological safety and learning behavior in work teams. Admin Sci Quart 1999;44:350–83.
26. Rowland P, Lising D, Sinclair L, et al. Team dynamics within quality improvement teams: a scoping review. Int J Qual Health Care 2018;30(6):416–22.
27. Nembhard IM, Edmondson AC. Making it safe: The effects of leader inclusiveness and professional status on psychological safety and improvement efforts in healthcare teams. J Organ Behav 2006;27:941–66.
28. Hammick M, Freeth D, Copperman J, et al. Being interprofessional. Cambridge (United Kingdom): Polity; 2009.
29. O'Leary D. Exploring the importance of team psychological safety in the development of two interprofessional teams. J Interprof Care 2016;30:29–34.
30. Lingard L, Espin S, Evans C, et al. The rules of the game: interprofessional collaboration on the intensive care unit team. Crit Care 2004;8(6):403–8.
31. Parsons ML, Batres C, Golightly-Jenkins C. Innovations in management: establishing team behavioral norms for a healthy workplace. Top Emerg Med 2006;28:113–9.
32. Parsons ML, Clark P, Marshall M, et al. Team behavioral norms: a shared vision for a healthy patient care workplace. Crit Care Nurs Q 2007;30(3):213–8.
33. Craigie FC, Hobbs R. Exploring the organizational culture of exemplary community health center practices. Fam Med 2004;36:733–8.
34. Orchard CA, King GA, Khalili H, et al. Assessment of Interprofessional Team Collaboration Scale (AITCS): development and testing of the instrument. J Contin Educ Health Prof 2012;32(1):58–67.
35. Orchard C, Pederson L, Read E, et al. Assessment of Interprofessional Team Collaboration Scale (AITCS): further testing and instrument revision. J Contin Educ Health Prof 2018;38(1):11–8.
36. Bosch M, Dijkstra R, Wensing M, et al. Organizational culture, team climate and diabetes care in small office–based practices. BMC Health Serv Res 2008;8:180.

37. Vachon B, LeBlanc J. Effectiveness of past and current critical incident analysis on reflective learning and practice change. Med Educ 2011;45(9):894–904.

38. Salas E, Klein C, King H, et al. Debriefing medical teams: 12 evidence-based best practices and tips. Jt Comm J Qual Patient Saf 2013;34(9):518–27.

39. Tannenbaum SI, Beard RL, Cerasoli CP. Conducting team debriefings that work: lessons from research and practice. Developing and enhancing teamwork in organizations: evidence-based best practices and guidelines. San Francisco: Jossey-Bass; 2013. p. 488–519.

40. Reyes DL, Tannenbaum SI, Salas E. Team development: the power of debriefing. People and Strategy 2018;41(2):46–51.

41. Leonard M, Graham S, Bonacum D. The human factor: the critical importance of effective teamwork and communication in providing safe care. Qual Saf Health Care 2004;13:i85–90.

42. Agency for Healthcare Research and Quality About TeamSTEPPS. 2019. Available at: https://www.ahrq.gov/teamstepps/about-teamstepps/index.html. Accessed June 14, 2018.

43. Parker AL, Forsythe LL, Kohlmorgen IK. TeamSTEPPS: an evidence-based approach to reduce clinical errors threatening safety in outpatient settings: an integrative review. J Healthc Risk Manag 2019;38:19–31.

44. Shams A, Ahmed M, Scalzitti NJ, et al. How does TeamSTEPPS affect operating room efficiency? Otolaryngol Head Neck Surg 2016;154(2):355–8.

45. Champagne H, Brennan E, Fildes D. TeamSTEPPS Training for obstetric and NICU multidisciplinary teams. JOGN Nurs 2019;48(3):S36.

46. Roman T, Abraham K, Dever K. TeamSTEPPS in long-term care—an academic partnership: Part II. J Contin Educ Nurs 2016;47(12):534–5.

47. Obenrader C, Broome M, Yap TL, et al. Changing team member perceptions by implementing TeamSTEPPS in an emergency department. J Emerg Nurs 2019; 45(1):31–7.

48. Thomas L, Galla C. Building a culture of safety through team training and engagement. BMJ Qual Saf 2013;22:425–34.

49. Armour Forse R, Bramble JD, McQuillan R. Team training can improve operating room performance. Surgery 2011;150:771–8.

50. Lee SH, Khanuja H, Blanding RJ, et al. Sustaining teamwork behaviours through reinforcement of TeamSTEPPS principles. J Patient Saf 2017. https://doi.org/10.1097/PTS.0000000000000414.

51. Institute for Healthcare Improvement (IHI). SBAR tool: situation-background-assessment-recommendation. Available at: http://www.ihi.org/resources/Pages/Tools/SBARToolkit.aspx. Accessed June 14, 2019.

52. Haig K, Sutton S, Whittington J. SBAR: a shared mental model for improving communication between clinicians. Jt Comm J Qual Saf 2006;32(3):167–75.

53. Kostoff M, Burkardt C, Winter A, et al. An interprofessional simulation using the SBAR communication tool. Am J Pharm Educ 2016;80(9):157.

54. Pope B, Rodzen L, Spross G. Raising the SBAR: how better communication improves patient outcomes. Nursing 2008;38(3):41–3.

55. Patterson K, Grenny J, McMillan R, et al. Crucial conversations: tools for talking when stakes are high. 2nd edition. New York: McGraw-Hill; 2011.

56. Cole J. Structural, organizational, and interpersonal factors influencing interprofessional collaboration on sexual assault response teams. J Interpers Violence 2018;33(17):2682–703.

57. Thomson K, Outram S, Gilligan C, et al. Interprofessional experiences of recent healthcare graduates: a social psychology perspective on the barriers to

effective communication, teamwork, and patient-centered care. J Interprof Care 2015;29(6):634–40.

58. Cooper-Duffy K, Eaker K. Effective team practices: Interprofessional contributions to communication issues with a parent's perspective. Am J Speech Lang Pathol 2017;26(2):181–92.

59. Lloyd J, Schneider J, Scales K, et al. Ingroup identity as an obstacle to effective multiprofessional and interprofessional teamwork: Findings from an ethnographic study of healthcare assistants in dementia care. J Interprof Care 2011;25:345–51.

60. Dow A, Zhu X, Sewell D, et al. Teamwork on the rocks: rethinking interprofessional practice as networking. J Interprof Care 2017;31:677–8.

61. Reeves S, Xyrichis A, Zwarenstein M. Teamwork, collaboration, coordination, and networking: Why we need to distinguish between different types of interprofessional practice. J Interprof Care 2018;32(1):1–3.

62. Canadian Interprofessional Health Collaborative. A National interprofessional competency framework. 2010. Available at: http://www.cihc.ca/files/CIHC_IPCompetencies_Feb1210.pdf. Accessed June 15, 2019.

Seeing Value in Physician Assistants

Ian W. Jones, MPAS, CCPA, PA-C

KEYWORDS

- Physician Assistants • PA • Value • Workforce economics
- Canadian physician assistants

KEY POINTS

- There is a disconnect between economic theory and healthcare delivery.
- Opportunity costs and cost-benefit analysis of role substitution within current hospital and community healthcare staffing models are seldom promoted.
- Attention focusing on using the most expensive health human resource, physicians, to their best extent, and changing policies to allow nonphysician providers to deliver medical services is required.
- The comparative advantage example and its real-world examples provide a route for improvement in value of healthcare delivery by professions.

INTRODUCTION

While sitting at a kitchen table negotiating the renewal of an employment contract, it occurred to the young Physician Assistant (PA) (Ian) that value was viewed differently by those in the room. The physician (Jim) was the owner/manager of the physician group contracted to provide emergency department services. The group paid an hourly wage to the PA. The physicians worked in a fee-for-service (FFS) environment where income related to patients seen and procedures performed. The emergency physicians pooled funds to pay the PA's wage. Every patient seen by physicians and PA required a record of the diagnosis and fee code. The PA worked evenings and weekends, reducing family time, but earning enough to support his lifestyle while paying student loans and mortgage. The physician group was requesting more holiday coverage and longer hours at a lower hourly rate. This demand for increased PA hours was generated by the hospital administrator, who paid the group a bonus for any reduction in the wait time. Wait times also affected patient satisfaction scores used in marketing efforts and quality improvement indicators by the hospital.

The author has no commercial interests to disclose.
The University of Manitoba, Max Rady College of Medicine, Winnipeg, Manitoba, Canada
E-mail address: Ian.Jones@umanitoba.ca
Twitter: @Ianjonesmpas (I.W.J.)

The negotiations continued with the PA showing his numbers, and the physician arguing costs. The owner's spouse walked into the kitchen, listened for a while, and interrupted: *"Jim, you need to keep Ian happy by limiting required hours, paying well for his services, and supporting him. Because for the first time in our marriage you are coming home on time. For years you stayed late to finish patient care. You didn't want to turn over cases to the next doctor. Let me sum it up for you, Jim, if Ian is not happy and leaves, you won't be happy. I will ensure you are not happy."*

The contract negotiations concluded to everyone's satisfaction.

> *Value defined as outcomes relative to costs encompasses efficiency. Cost reduction without regard to the outcomes achieved is dangerous and self-defeating, leading to false 'savings' and potentially limiting effective care.*
> —*Michael Porter, Harvard Business Review, "What Is Value in Health Care?"[1]*

Value, adequately understood, highlights patient centeredness as a critical dimension of quality and the burdens of treatment (for patients) and care delivery (for providers) as important aspects of cost. The error, then, lies not in pursuing value too far but in not pursuing it far enough.[2]

HOW DO WE DETERMINE THE VALUE OF A PHYSICIAN ASSISTANT IN HEALTHCARE?

PAs are ultimately related to value, dollars, and needs. Business journals define value as the return related to the investment cost. Values in philosophy are standards or ideals with which to evaluate actions, people, things, or situations. Beauty, honesty, justice, peace, and generosity are all examples of values that many people endorse. The essence of economics is the three underlying principles of scarcity, efficiency, and sovereignty. The medical concept of value reflects needs, wishes, preferences, and the ethics of providing value-centric patient care. Economists do not define these principles, but the basic principles of human behavior exist regardless of market economies or planned economies. If health and wellness are scarce and affects the quality of life, it has value. Few people want to wait for service or wait to have care. People also, in general, seek self-determination, the right to choose options and their paths. Human behavior ultimately defines what determines an object or person's value.[3–6]

Value plays a crucial role in healthcare systems. The definition of value varies according to the perspective or viewpoints of physicians, patients, other providers, payers, or system administrators. Medical practice innovations and the increasing attention to patient-centeredness have introduced value-based medicine into current health systems approaches.[7]

A definition of value in healthcare provided by Dr Steven E. Wegner of the Centres for Medicare and Medicare Services states that value equals quality over costs. The concept describes quality measures whereby the cost of providing and addressing healthcare processes, outcomes, patient perceptions, organizational structure, and system's cost are measured by association with healthcare outcomes and meeting the goals for quality healthcare. These goals include effective, safe, efficient, patient-centered, equitable, and timely care. Most of the suggestions are process measures with limited patient input. In essence, what does it cost to make things better?[8]

Another conceptual approach in measuring value outcomes uses a time-driven activity-based costing (ABC) method.[8,9] Time-driven ABC limits data needed, requiring estimates of committed resources and their cost, and unit times for performing activities. The accounting measure is simplified as what was done, how much did it cost, and how long did it take.

From the patient's viewpoint, the definition of value may simply be, "What am I getting, am I going to get better, and how much did it cost?"

According to the New Economics Foundation, social return of investment captures social value by translating outcomes into financial values. Does the investment in services or support to the economy provide a tangible and intangible value to the community? The evaluation of PA's values considers the social return provided not just to patients but also to the physician workforce.

The classic article, "What Is Value in Health Care?," was published in the *Harvard Business Review* in 2010. Written by Michael Porter, it indicated that value must consider the end user or customer or, in healthcare, the patient. Value for patients requires a determination of the rewards for all those in the system. Results matter, not inputs, and outcomes achieved, not the numbers or the range of services delivered. The challenge is shifting of viewpoint from volume to value issues. Quality measures abound, but the question of whether people are happier and healthier is the real measure and goal.[1]

A broad consensus on the meaning of "value" is still lacking. Patients, physicians, policymakers, and other healthcare professionals have different ideas on which component of value plays a prominent role.[10] Recognizing that shared clinical decision making with patient empowerment is a central concept of value, and different paradigms of healthcare systems embrace different meanings of value. There is no single definitive standard or widely accepted definition of value. There is even less academic work addressing the value of a PA to the practice and the physician employer.

THE PHYSICIAN ASSISTANT

PAs appear as an underexplored addition to the healthcare system. PAs receive generalist training, have condensed educational programs, and receive proportionately lower salary scales. The MD-PA team collaboration generates flexibility and responsiveness that supplements and improves efficiency within healthcare systems.[11–16]

The traditional hierarchy approach to healthcare delivery places physicians and nurses as the primary deliverers of healthcare. Despite the increase and benefits of interprofessional health teams, alternatives providers, such as PAs, nurse practitioners (NPs), midwives, and other professional clinicians, are overlooked in health resource strategies. The current system neglects the opportunity costs of existing professionals by not effectively investigating alternative delivery models. Although dynamic and continuously shifting in response to innovation in technology, the healthcare system tends to miss the possibilities of using the services and talent of nonphysicians or nurses. Forward-thinking management structures are often sidelined in policy debates, placing new technologies and scientific discoveries ahead of human resources.[17–20]

The healthcare system focuses on providing medical care with an emphasis on disease management by professionals. Consider how a medical provider such as a PA optimizes healthcare.

The PA role is the authorized task substitution of medical acts traditionally reserved for physicians. The PA's value is efficiency and effectiveness and within the economic realities of the healthcare system. PAs are medically educated to function as generalist clinicians in primary care provider roles in medical service to communities, or hospital-based roles, such as in-patient, emergency, or surgery. The PA's education and authorization allow them to function in any clinical setting within a formalized agreement with physicians. When used to their full capacity, or scope of practice, PAs supplement and support physicians in a clinician role, increasing services and patient's access to quality medical care, and improving efficiencies in medical service delivery. Ultimately, the PA's value is determined through the lenses of those looking and asking what is needed, whether individually or collectively, and depending on whether the viewer is patient, physician, or an administrator.

The Cost of a Physician Centric Model

One of the most fundamental concepts in economics, comparative advantage provides a simple way to highlight the effectiveness of PAs as a cost-effective healthcare practitioner. Comparative advantage is a way of looking at a cost-benefit production choice between two somewhat similar groups with different wages and productivity. Comparative advantage is traditionally used to understand international trade but also applied to the example of PAs and physicians.

A medical provider with the comparative advantage provides medical care for a cheaper cost per patient than their alternative. The benefits of using a provider with less education, although still qualified and competent, make acquiring goods or services faster and less costly. Shorter length of education costs less to the system and individual learners (**Fig. 1**). Being less expensive, more readily available, and approachable outweighs the disadvantages of a narrower education and clinical leaning experience. Saving educational time by removing specialized knowledge in topics such as embryology or perhaps genetics allows a focus on more primary care common concerns. The disadvantage is that medicine is becoming more sophisticated, and introduction of genomic pharmacology may change primary clinical practice in the future.

Comparative advantage is used intuitively every day. Some of the questions are as follows: Can time spent by a neurosurgeon or cardiac surgeon in a clinic performing patient's admission histories and physical examinations be better used in surgery?

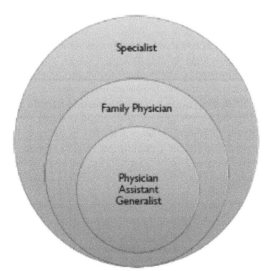

Fig. 1. Educational representative overlap of specialist MD, family practice (generalist) MD, and PA generalist practice and education.

Can another professional provide the quality of history and physical examinations at a lower unit or hourly cost? If suturing a wound or investigation of abdominal pain by a PA allows more experienced critical thinking to be applied elsewhere, there is a system gain. A highly educated and trained surgeon may be more efficient at processing patient intakes than the administrative assistant at the front desk, but this is not an efficient use of the surgeon's time. The physician may see more patients than the PA in the clinic over the same time, but the surgeon or physician earns several times more per hour than the alternatives. The goal of a comparative advantage analysis is to find the most cost-effective combination of health professionals to provide the best quality healthcare for patients.

Physicians' specialized knowledge is acquired through years of education, including undergraduate and postgraduate medical education. Subsequently, physician remuneration is higher than other healthcare alternatives.[21-27] According to the Canadian Institute for Health Information in 2017, the total gross clinical payments to Canada's 86,644 physicians reached C$26.4 billion in 2016 to 2017, a 2.8% increase over the previous year, an average gross income of C$304,695. Gross income is an intermediate earnings figure before consideration of expenses, and net income is the final amount of profit or loss after expenses.[22,23,28-30]

The PA's generalist medical training leads to a career focus on clinical practice and developing further knowledge in a medical specialty over time. Attainment of additional job knowledge and skills is a design characteristic of the profession that improves the efficiency of PA services. High-quality care of a PA costs one-third to one-half the salary of a physician with the scope of practice estimated at 70% to 80% of defined general practice productivity.[31-34] There is a range of numbers reflecting estimated productivity, the nature of the practice, experiences the practitioner brings, and community demographics. Economic modeling is a challenge to quantify the exact measurement. For those uncomfortable with the substitution of a nonphysician provider for traditional physician tasks, it is a challenge to change perspective. PAs manage patients within their scope of practice by working collaboratively with physicians. The integral members of healthcare teams support and extend physician services, not replace them.

Comparative advantage analysis quantifies the time required to perform a specific medical task, such as biopsies, laceration repair, or clinical consultation, assuming that a procedure performed by a physician and a PA are effectively the same. The time for procedure will range from no time at all to "X" number of minutes. Time spent depends on experience and skills and factors the hourly wage of the medical personnel in question. Assume that consultation time will decrease over time as the PA becomes more experienced in a particular task. Comparing the physician's cost-per-procedure to the PA's cost time and an hourly rate for the procedure provides a comparative advantage analysis. The model is simple but overwhelmingly supported by empirical tests and the labor market. The expansion of PAs in the United States demonstrates that quality of care is equal.[33-36]

For example, if it takes 10 minutes for a physician to complete a clinical consultation and the PA 15 minutes to do the same consultation, and the physician remuneration is $120 per hour and the PA's remuneration is $45, the relative cost would be $20 per physician consult, and $13 per PA consult. The PA-physician team treats 1.42 patients for the same cost as a solo physician. It is likely more cost-effective for the PA to perform the clinical consultations, freeing the physician for other patients or duties.

The comparative advantage exercise reflected in **Fig. 2** indicates procedures optimally performed by a PA or physiotherapist found to the left and below the dotted line and for those to the right by family physicians and above by specialist physicians like surgeons. The curved line represents cost and experience curve, with the red dashed

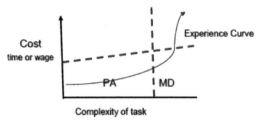

Fig. 2. Comparative advantage diagram.

line a breakeven point for PA and physicians being equally qualified to perform a task at the same cost.

PAs and NPs cost less and deliver care comparable to family physicians. There is an argument that having one individual that can do 100% of a job makes sense, but not if the cost is three times more than the alternative needed. A PA or NP cannot match the skills and experiences of a neurosurgeon or transplant specialist. The skills needed for taking histories or performing a physical examination, identifying the medical issues or the management of common ailments, do not require the same level of surgical expertise.

THE PA's COST TO A MEDICAL PRACTICE

This calculation is an estimated guide to provide the perspective of value and actual cost calculations:

If the PA annual compensation + benefits	= $100,000 and assuming a
supervisory cost calculation of 10%	+ $10,000 (MD reimbursement + insurance)
Moreover, factor in the occupancy space costs	+ $10,000 (an examination room)
Also, pay for the technology support	+ $5000
The annual costs of a PA	=$125,000

Out of 365 days in a year, a PA in an outpatient clinic will work approximately 224 days a year, or approximately 18.7 days per month, accounting for weekends, vacation, and statutory holidays. In an 8-hour day, the PA typically has some nonproductive time for lunch, meetings, or paid education, leaving approximately 6.5 hours per day to see patients. Therefore, the actual hourly cost is approximately $85.85 per clinical hour. (The total cost of $125,000, divided by the total hours per year of 224 days × 6.5 hours = 1456 hours per year.) The PA is an expensive employee, but still only half that of a physician costing $188.87/clinical hour ($275,000 [average] ÷ 1456 = $188.87/h, based on the cost of a family or emergency MD provided by the Canadian Institute for Health Information.)

Using a medical team rather than a single doctor with support staff has been shown to be a useful model for healthcare services.[33–36] A medical team focuses on a multilayered approach to healthcare with medical professionals of varying levels of academic qualifications. A specialist physician provides the medical care for the most challenging procedures, such as a neurosurgical clipping of a cerebral aneurysm, whereas more generalist professionals, such as family doctors or surgical nurses, perform less complex procedures, such as biopsies, wound repair, or surgical closures.

Utilization of PAs increases the generalist services provided to the clinic, ward, surgical suite, or patient follow-up. Consultation with the specialist, as required, uses time efficiently. An excellent example of team-based medicine is the shared care concept in mental health, where social workers, counselors, psychologists, psychiatric NPs, and psychiatrists provide services through vertical integration. Basic levels of healthcare can be provided for a broader demographic and patient population, whereas a smaller number of specialists perform the more specialized procedure or service. A PA often functions as the intermediary within these healthcare teams, serving as a bridge between initial intake and more complex medical procedure of physicians.

PHYSICIAN PERSPECTIVE ON PHYSICIAN ASSISTANT VALUE

Having a PA work with me is akin to finding that perfect Ballroom Dance partner, someone who gets it. That moment when everything comes together; movements don't require talking; they just happen. Having a partner who knows what has to be done and what comes next. That is the sense I get from working with my PA.
—Personal Email Communication with John Embil, MD, FRCPC,
Professor, Director of Health Sciences Centre, Infection Prevention and
Control Unit, May, 2019

As part of an ongoing quality assurance study by the University of Manitoba Masters of Physician Assistant Studies, an electronic survey sought to gather physicians' perspectives of PA value (May 2019). The survey was distributed to physicians identified as employing or supervising PAs in Manitoba, based on program records. Twenty physicians responded from the list of 72 contacted, representing a response rate of 27.7%. Three of the physician respondents employed a PA for less than a year, 85% or 16 physicians employed a PA for more than 2 years, with 36.84% of the total employed a PA for longer than 5 years. One did not indicate. Eighteen of the 20 responding physicians indicated being in practice for more than 5 years, 14 for more than 10 years. The physician respondents represented surgery 40%, family medicine 20%, emergency 15%, hospitalist role 5%, 10% from a mixed specialty clinic, 5% from pediatrics, and 5% other. This breakdown is reflective of the known employment patterns for Winnipeg PAs, with underrepresentation from psychiatry and rural communities. In order to ensure confidentiality, the survey did not gather any personal identifying information or Internet addresses of respondents. The nature of the specialty was limited to broad categories.

Manitoba PAs have employment in 32 medical or surgical specialties. The 20% (n = 4) of PAs supervised were from the Canadian Armed Forces, 85% (n = 17) from University of Manitoba, and one PA was American educated.

One physician or 5% of respondents indicated they were not likely to recommend hiring a PA, whereas 95% (19) were likely or extremely likely to recommend hiring a PA to a friend or colleague. Overall satisfaction with the PAs' medical knowledge was 75%, with 20% somewhat satisfied. Related to patient care provided by the PAs, 95% indicated extreme satisfaction or very satisfied, whereas one was neither satisfied nor dissatisfied.

When asked about personal satisfaction since hiring a PA, 90% of the physicians indicated positive enjoyment, with increased satisfaction with their career. Words identified after addition of a PA to the practice included "less stress, better life, more relaxed at work, increased productivity, good value for money, and improved my career." The one detractor said, "never again."

The 85% (n = 18/20) of the physicians rated the value of having a PA working with them as very or extremely valuable; one indicated somewhat valuable, and one indicated not at all. When rating the value for money for a PA, 85% indicated above average or excellent value. Fifty percent of responding physicians indicated that if they were able to generate revenue from services provided by the PA, they would employ a PA directly. One physician indicted they would not. In Manitoba, 90% of PAs are salaried employees of the Regional Health Authorities. Manitoba Health Insurance is a single-payer system. A few projects are piloting FFS models.

The response for the value of PAs brought to Manitoba Health Care included honesty and respect (78.95%), improved access (73%), excellence in care (63.1%), better workplace communication (78.95%), better patient safety (73.68%), better teamwork (84.21%), accountability (73.68%), efficiency (73.68%), decreased stress (42.11%), and better communication with patients (57.89%).

In the questions answered, there was one detractor who was consistently unhappy with their PA. The individual's responses indicated a subspecialty practice with a new graduate PA who did not have prior clinical experience. Comments provided indicated that the lack of prior experience was detrimental to their subspecialty practice. Not having clinical experience is shared with 80% of the graduates of the Manitoba program and in most undergraduate medical students. The University of Manitoba prepares graduates as generalist medical practitioners for primary care and community hospital roles. It appears that the hiring process was flawed in this case, and expectations were not appropriately addressed.

Most physicians in Winnipeg appear delighted with the quality and value PAs brought to their practice environment and personal lives. In days whereby stress and burnout are common topics in the professional journals and faculty meetings of physicians, this is a significant finding.

CURRENT FUNDING MODELS

PAs funding is through salary, the FFS, and capitated models. In the United States and Canada, FFS models are insurance-based reimbursements for evaluation services, management of care, and the procedures performed. FFS is a payment model for services separately reimbursed at an assigned tariff or rate. FFS models are rare in Canadian PA practice. Salary models are hourly or annual payment models for services provided under contract to an employer. Job descriptions assigning duties are the most common Canadian model known to the author. Capitation payments are payments agreed upon in a capitated contract by a health insurance company and a medical provider. There are prearranged monthly payments received by a physician, clinic, or hospital per each patient enrolled in a health plan, or per capita.[37] Health maintenance organizations and preferred provider organizations administer the most common types of managed care health insurance plans using per capita payment models.

There are hybrids and variations for each of the primary models. Alternated funding models combine several components, linking nonmedical services such as teaching or administration to reimbursement. Pay-for-performance has the potential to help improve the quality of care if aligned with the goals of medical professionalism, but little evidence exists on its effectiveness. These initiatives provide incentives for a specific element of a single disease or condition. However, it may neglect the complexity of care for the whole patient, especially the elderly patient with multiple chronic conditions.[37]

PA funding models must consider the close working relationship between the PA and the supervising physician. Political and financial pressures complicate compensation for the oversight of another health professional, and a one-size-fits-all approach will not work. Provincial rules of application that govern physician billing practices are the primary stumbling block to addressing PA compensation. Until physicians can either bill for the work done by the PA, or the PA can bill for their patient encounters, PAs cannot work to their full scope of practice. Physicians are therefore forced to either replicate the work already done by the PA or risk violating the rules of application.

SUMMARY: WHY IS THIS IMPORTANT?

There is a disconnect between economic theory and healthcare delivery. Opportunity costs and cost-benefit analysis of role substitution within current hospital and community healthcare staffing models are seldom promoted. Attention focusing on using the most expensive health human resource, physicians, to their best extent, and changing policies to allow nonphysician providers to deliver medical services is required. The comparative advantage example and its real-world examples provide a route for improvement in value of healthcare delivery by professions.

Can PAs provide high-quality, patient-centric care using a lower cost approach? Yes; however, effectiveness, efficiency, and economy are all interrelated. Determining the PA's value to the health system requires a broader context than a purely financial approach. Considering the social implications of efficiency and effectiveness means looking at what people value, or the human factor. The political and economic realities are essential considerations. Patients have a stake in the quality and value of care provided. In democracies, people vote for governments, and those governments fund and design health systems and medical services, whether FFS, salary, or other models.

Value has different meanings to different people, related to their roles. A healthy accountant sees unit cost per output or throughput. If the accountant becomes a patient, perspective shifts to determining what is needed to get healthy and back to work or family. Happiness is vital to everyone, and frequently discussed is achieving the right balance at work and home. Health and happiness are values deemed necessary to patients, physicians, and PAs. Physicians and PAs provide value to the health system regardless of the metric used. Seeing the value in PAs means looking for more than the cost and return on investments but the effect and impact on others.

REFERENCES

1. Porter ME, Teisberg EO. Redefining healthcare: creating value-based competition on results. Boston: Harvard Business School Press; 2006.
2. Starr SR, Agrawal N, et al. Mayo Clinic – Letter to the Editor Academic Medicine, Vol. 94, No. 6. 2019.
3. Pittman TS, Zeigler KR. Basic Human Needs; Personal Motivational System. In: Kruglanski AW, Higgins ET, editors. Social Psychology: Handbook of Basic Principles. New York: Guilford Press; 2007.
4. Zeckhauser R, Eliastam M. The productivity potential of the physician assistant. J Hum Resour 1974;9(1):95–116.
5. Marzorati C, Pravettoni G. Value as the key concept in the healthcare system: how it has influenced medical practice and clinical decision-making processes. J Multidiscip Healthc 2017;10:101–6.
6. Ikerd J. The three economic principles of sustainability posted: Feb 25, 2013. CSRwire Talkback Blog. 2013. Available at: https://www.csrwire.com/blog/posts/733-the-three-economic-principles-of-sustainability. Accessed March, 2019.
7. Ken Lee KH, Matthew Austin J, Pronovost PJ. Developing a measure of value in healthcare. Value Health 2016;19(4):323–5.

8. Wegner SE. Measuring Value in Health Care: The Times, They Are A Changin'. N C Med J 2016;77(4):276–8.

9. Liu N, D'Aunno T. The productivity and cost-efficiency of models for involving nurse practitioners in primary care: a perspective from queuing analysis. Health Serv Res 2012;47(2):594–613.

10. Snyder L, Neubauer RL, for the American College of Physicians Ethics, Professionalism and Human Rights Committee. Pay-for-performance principles that promote patient-centered care: an ethics manifesto. Ann Intern Med 2007;147:792–4.

11. Hooker RS. Federally employed physician assistants. Mil Med 2008;173:895–9.

12. Hooker RS. Physician assistants in the Canadian forces. Mil Med 2003;168:948–50.

13. Hooker R. Physician assistants and nurse practitioners: the United States experience. Med J Aust 2006;185:4–7.

14. Hooker R, Everette C. The contributions of physician assistants in primary care systems. Health Soc Care Community 2012;20(1):20–31.

15. Jones IW, St-Pierre W. Physician Assistants in Canada. Journal of the American Academy of Physician Assistants 2014;27(3):11–3.

16. Jones I, Ives R, Burrows K, et al. A perspective on the economic sustainability of the physician assistant profession in Canada. JCANPA.ca 2018;1:1.

17. Kernick DP. Introduction to health economics for the medical practitioner. Postgrad Med J 2003;79:147–50.

18. Russell LB, Sinha A. Strengthening Cost-Effectiveness Analysis for Public Health Policy. Am J Prev Med 2016;50(5 Suppl 1):S6–12.

19. Hooker RS, Everett CM. The contributions of physician assistants in primary care systems. Health & Social Care in the Community 2012;20:20–31.

20. Bourgeault IL, Mulvale G. Collaborative healthcare teams in Canada and the USA: confronting the structural embeddedness of medical dominance. Health Sociol Rev 2006;15(5):481–95.

21. Canadian Institute for Health Information, The regulation and supply of nurse practitioners in Canada: 2006 Update. Available at: http://www.publications.gc.ca/site/eng/293146/publication.html.

22. Canadian Institute for Health Information, Experiences with primary healthcare in Canada, June 2009. Available at: https://secure.cihi.ca/free_products/cse_phc_aib_en.pdf.

23. Cawley JF. Physician assistant supply and demand. JAAPA 2005;18(8):11–2.

24. Legler CF, Cawley JF, Fenn WH. Physician assistants: education, practice and global interest. Medical Teacher 2007;29(1):e22–5.

25. Conference Board of Canada: lack of sustainable funding a barrier to physician assistant employment in Canada. 2017. Available at: http://www.conferenceboard.ca/press/newsrelease/17-09-13/lack_of_sustainable_funding_a_barrier_to_physician_assistant_employment_in_canada.asp. Accessed March, 2019

26. Grimes K, Prada G. Value of Physician Assistants: Understanding the Role of Physician Assistants Within Health Systems. The Conference Board of Canada. Available at: https://www.conferenceboard.ca/e-library/abstract.aspx?did=8107.

27. Dineen K. Responsibility and collaboration in health team care. Virtual Mentor 2009;11(3):247–52.

28. Gerrie B, Holbrook E. The evolutionary role of physician assistants across the United States, Canada, and the United Kingdom. Int J Exerc Sci 2013;6(1):1–8.

29. Morgan A, Perri ND, Shah JS, et al. Impact of physician assistant care on office visit resource use in the United States. Health Serv Res 2008;43(5 Pt 2):1906–22.

30. Grzybicki DM, Sullivan PJ, Oppy JM, et al. The economic benefit for family/general medicine practices employing physician assistants. Am J Manag Care 2002; 8(7):613–20.
31. Woodmansee D, Hooker R. Physician Assistants Working in the Department of Veterans Affairs. JAAPA 2010;23(11):41–4.
32. Larson EH, Hart LG, Ballweg R. National estimates of physician assistant productivity. J Allied Health 2001;30(3):146–52.
33. Kurtzman ET, Barnow BS, et al. A comparison of nurse practitioners, physician assistants, and primary care physicians' patterns of practice and quality of care in health centers. Med Care 2017;55:615–22.
34. Cawley JF. Physician Assistants and Their Role in Primary Care. Virtual Mentor 2012;14(5):411–4.
35. Hooker RS. Physician assistants and nurse practitioners: the United States experience. Med J Aust 2006;185(1):4–7.
36. Huckabee M, Wheeler D. Defining leadership training for physician assistant education. J Physician Assist Educ 2008;19(1):24–8.
37. Porter ME, Kaplan RS. How to Pay for Health Care. Harvard Business Review 2016. Available at: https://hbr.org/2016/07/how-to-pay-for-health-care. Accessed May, 2019.

FURTHER READINGS

The American Academy of Physician Assistants. Third party reimbursements for PAs. 2017. Available at: https://www.aapa.org/.

Competency-Based Medical Education for Physician Assistants

The Development of Competency-Based Medical Education and Competency Frameworks in the United States and Canada

Sharona Kanofsky, PA-C, CCPA, MScCH

KEYWORDS

- Competency-based medical education • Physician Assistants
- Physician Assistants education • Competency frameworks

KEY POINTS

- Competency-based medical education (CBME) is currently the gold standard of physician assistant education in the United States, Canada, and around the world.
- CBME emphasizes observable, standardized outcomes and flexibility in the timing of attainment of competence.
- CBME was first developed for graduate medical education in the United States and Canada in the late 1990s and quickly spread to undergraduate medical education, physician assistant education, and many other health professions around the world.

Traditional forms of education have a fixed time with variable outcome, whereas CBE has a fixed outcome with variable time.
—Robert Englander, University of Minnesota Medical School, "Competence by Design." Available at: http://www.royalcollege.ca/rcsite/cbd/rationale-why-cbd-e

INTRODUCTION

Competency-based medical education (CBME) is the current gold standard of physician assistant (PA) education in the United States, Canada, and around the world. CBME was first developed for graduate medical education in the United States and Canada in the late 1990s. It quickly spread to undergraduate physician education,

Department of Family and Community Medicine, Physician Assistant Program, 263 McCaul Street, 3rd Floor, Toronto, Ontario, M5T 1W7, Canada
E-mail address: sharona.kanofsky@utoronto.ca

Physician Assist Clin 5 (2020) 91–107
https://doi.org/10.1016/j.cpha.2019.08.005
2405-7991/20/© 2019 Elsevier Inc. All rights reserved.

physicianassistant.theclinics.com

PA education, and many other health professions in these countries and globally. CBME, and the related competency frameworks, are now well-established, useful models for healthcare education and practice, and they will be here for a long time to come.

In this article, we explore the development of CBME and the evolution of the competency frameworks, first in physician education, and then for the PA profession in the United States and Canada. We briefly compare these competency frameworks and consider the context accounting for some of the differences between them.

During the early years of its implementation, CBME and competency frameworks have demonstrated some limitations, particularly in the application of these theoretic frameworks to the real-world setting of clinical teaching and learning. We consider some developments in CBME that attempt to bridge the gap between theory and practice. These include Milestones, Entrustable Professional Activities (EPAs), and Competence by Design.

As with any popular trend, it is also useful to look at CBME with a critical lens. We consider which values may potentially be overemphasized, and which ones underemphasize. We end by exploring some of the common critiques of CBME that have emerged during the height of its popularity, in an effort to better understand the value and potential pitfalls of CBME and competency frameworks.

COMPETENCY-BASED EDUCATION AND PRACTICE

CBME has its roots in the teacher education reform of the 1960s. In teacher education, the transition from traditional educational models to a performance-based model emphasized learner achievement, demonstrated by observable outcomes.[1] In CBME, these outcomes are categorized within specific areas of competency, based on the desired educational outcomes of the program.

Competency is described as "a complex set of behaviors built on the components of knowledge, skills, and attitudes," and *competence* is described as personal ability.[2(p362)] Competencies can be demonstrated and observed through their application. For physicians, PAs, and other healthcare professionals, the application of competence is generally demonstrated in clinical practice and in related professional activities.

Competency-based education has a number of identifiable features[1]: competencies are derived directly from the expected roles of the professional (ie, the specific roles of the teacher, physician, PA, etc.); assessment is directly related to demonstration by the learner (and observation by faculty) of the acceptable standards of achievement within that area of competence; and performance is the primary source of evidence for attainment of competence, although some value is also placed on demonstration of knowledge. The criteria for demonstration and observation of these learning outcomes are clearly established before learning. The learner's progress through the program of study is determined by achievement of competence, which can be variable among learners, rather than the length of the program, which is typically fixed.[1]

Comparing CBME with traditional forms of structure- or process-based medical education, some of the key differences include the following:[2] In CBME, the emphasis of the curriculum and the goal of the educational encounter is on observable outcomes and the application of knowledge, whereas traditional curricula emphasize learning the content and acquisition of knowledge. The process of learning in CBME is focused on the learner's specific needs, whereas traditional education focuses more on delivery of content by the teacher. The path of learning in CBME is nonhierarchical, with horizontal interaction between teacher and learning (ie, "a guide on the side"), whereas traditional education is hierarchical, with the teacher imparting content to the learner (ie, "the sage on the stage"). Assessment in CBME ideally uses multiple objective measures, with tools that are authentic and simulate the real-world setting in which the competency will be applied, whereas traditional assessments typically use fewer, less objective tools to measure competence by proxy, such as written tests or essays to demonstrate knowledge removed from its application. Emphasis in CBME assessment is on formative feedback, whereas the emphasis in traditional education is on summative feedback. Overall, assessment of competence in CBME is criterion referenced, meaning that the individual learner is assessed in relation to predetermined standards of competence, whereas traditional assessments are often norm referenced, meaning that learners are compared with their peers, rather than objective standards. Importantly, in CBME, the timing of program completion is ideally variable, with different learners achieving competence at varying rates, whereas traditional education is based on a fixed program length.[2(p362)] This element of variable timing is one of the more challenging aspects of CBME to operationalize, owing to the logistical challenges of customizing program length for each learner's needs (**Table 1**).

Carraccio and colleagues[2(p365)] describe four steps for implementing CBME. The first step is to identify the desired competencies (such as the six domains of the ACGME competencies or the seven roles in the CanMEDS framework). The second step is to identify the components and outcome expectancy for each of the competencies as a series of benchmarks or performance indicators. The third step is developing an assessment strategy to ensure learners are achieving the various components third is and assessment. Finally, there must be dedicated faculty development for faculty involved in teaching within the CBME curriculum.

Table 1
A comparison of the elements of structure- and process-based versus competency-based educational programs

Variable	Educational Program	
	Structure and Process Based	Competency Based
Driving force for curriculum	Content—knowledge acquisition	Outcome—knowledge application
Driving force for process	Teacher	Learner
Path of teaming	Hierarchical (teacher ⇒ student)	Nonhierarchical (teacher ⇔ student)
Responsibility for content	Teacher	Student and teacher
Goal of educational encounter	Knowledge acquisition	Knowledge application
Typical assessment tool	Single subjective measure	Multiple objective measures ("evaluation portfolio")
Assessment tool	Proxy	Authentic (mimics real tasks of profession)
Setting for evaluation	Removed (gestalt)	"In the trenches" (direct observation)
Evaluation	Norm referenced	Criterion referenced
Timing of assessment	Emphasis on summative	Emphasis on formative
Program completion	Fixed time	Variable time

From Carraccio C , Wolfsthal SD, Englander R, et al. Shifting paradigms: from Flexner to competencies. Acad Med. 2002 May;77(5):361-7.

WHY COMPETENCY-BASED MEDICAL EDUCATION IN MEDICAL EDUCATION?

In the late 20th century, medical education and practice came under social scrutiny from several directions. Some of the forces included attitudes of consumerism in the public, with a shifting attitude of medical service as a consumer product; increasing government regulations; increasing healthcare costs and worsening financial constraints within the healthcare system; increasing availability of health information online; increasing risk of medical litigation; and an explosion in medical technology and knowledge.[3–5] In response to these societal pressures, the medical professions in the United States and Canada recognized the need to become more socially accountable and transparent, particularly in the standards and expectations for physicians and medical trainees. This situation eventually led to a major renewal in medical education and practice. Similar trends developed globally, but here we focus on the United States and Canada.

COMPETENCY FRAMEWORKS

Perhaps the most dramatic innovation of this renewal was the establishment of competency-based education as the standard for medical education (and eventually for other health professions education) and the related development of the now ubiquitous competency frameworks. The shift toward transparent expectations, objective standards, observable competency-based outcomes, and the identification of physician roles led naturally toward the development of frameworks to organize and categorize these competencies.

Typically, a competency framework is composed of a group of general competency domains or roles. These are the major categories in the framework and, taken together, make up a compliment of attributes that reflect a well-rounded, competent professional. Each of these domains (or roles) is further divided and subdivided into specific outcomes—knowledge, skills, or attitudes—that can be observed and assessed. These outcomes form the basis for educational programming, such as curriculum developments, assessment strategies, accreditation, and standard setting.

ACCREDITATION COUNCIL OF GRADUATE MEDICAL EDUCATION OUTCOMES PROJECT IN THE UNITED STATES

The Accreditation Council of Graduate Medical Education (ACGME) implemented CBME for American graduate medical education, introducing the first general competencies framework in 1998, and eventually developing this framework further, in the Outcomes Project of 2001. Six domains of competence were identified that, combined, reflect a competent physician, equipped with a complete skillset to care for patients and work effectively and efficiently within the healthcare system. The six ACGME general competency domains (developed with the American Board of Medical Specialties) are (1) patient care, (2) medical knowledge, (3) practice-based learning and improvement, (4) interpersonal and communication skills, (5) professionalism, and (6) systems-based practice.[6]

Each of these domains includes several constituent components. For example, patient care includes (1) communicating effectively, demonstrating caring and respectful behavior, and (2) gathering essential and accurate information. Medical knowledge includes (1) obtaining biomedical, clinical, social-behavioral, and epidemiologic knowledge, and (2) demonstrating investigatory and analytical thinking.[6]

Overall, this theoretic model for organizing graduate medical education was successful. However, there were some practical challenges to implementing this model, which are addressed elsewhere in this article.

EDUCATING FUTURE PHYSICIANS OF ONTARIO AND CanMEDS IN CANADA

In Canada, a similar need to respond to the above-mentioned societal pressures led to the Educating Future Physicians of Ontario (EFPO) project, and later to the Can-MEDS Competency Framework. In 1986, Ontario physicians went on strike over an impending legislation to curtail extra billing, a practice that allowed physicians to charge patients beyond the fees for medical services covered by the provincial government health insurance plan. The public did not support the striking physicians and this episode became a public relations defeat for the physician community; the medical profession's reputation was tarnished. Physicians and educators collaborated to address the growing gap between the medical profession and the public.[7] EFPO was a collaborative project in the early 1990s among the five medical schools in Ontario.

Similar to the ACGME Outcomes Project, the EFPO sought to update Canadian medical education to meet societal views of the competent physician.[8] Gathering input about notions of a competent physician from many stakeholders, including education experts, physicians, medical students and the public, EFPO distilled their findings into eight physician roles.

In 1996, the Royal College of Physicians and Surgeons of Canada (RCPSC), building on the findings of EFPO, developed and introduced the CanMEDS framework (**Fig. 1**) for graduate medical education, which outlined the essential competencies of a physician. Over time, the CanMEDS framework gained popularity and was eventually applied to the RCPSC's accreditation, assessment, and continued professional development standards.

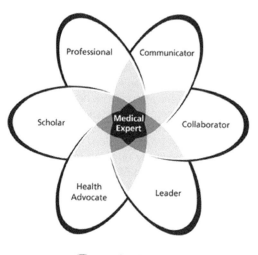

Fig. 1. CanMEDS Diagram (Copyright © 2015 The Royal College of Physicians and Surgeons of Canada. http://www.royalcollege.ca/rcsite/canmeds/canmeds-framework-e. Reproduced with permission.)

The CanMEDS framework, revised in 2005 and 2015, was soon adopted and adapted for use at multiple levels of medical education, including curriculum development, assessment, program accreditation, professional certification, and continued professional development. CanMEDS further spread to many other healthcare professions in Canada and globally. CanMEDS was originally an abbreviation for the *Canadian Medical Education Directives for Specialists*. With the broad deployment of the framework, the name CanMEDS is no longer used as an acronym, but is now a standalone name. The global impact of CanMEDS on medicine and other healthcare professions cannot be overstated.

CanMEDS identifies seven physician roles that together reflect a holistically competent physician. These seven roles are (1) Medical Expert, (2) Communicator, (3) Collaborator, (4) Leader (manager before the 2015 update), (5) Health Advocate, (6) Scholar, and (7) Professional.

The Royal College's CanMEDS framework is depicted in fig. 1. In this venn diagram, the central role of the physician is the medical expert role. There are areas of overlap between the central role of Medical Expert and the surrounding roles. The diagram implies that the central role of the physician is as Medical Expert. This is the knowledge and skillset that distinguishes the medical professional from the lay person. However, the diagram also indicates that this central role relies upon the support of each of the other roles evenly distributed around the center. The overlap between each of the roles in the diagram demonstrates that the roles are intertwined and interdependent. Together, these roles represent a competent, well-rounded physician.

COMPETENCIES FOR THE PHYSICIAN ASSISTANT PROFESSION

The PA professional organizations responded to the growth of competency-based models of education and practice by developing a competency framework for the PA profession. In addition to responding to the growing trend in healthcare education, this effort was intended to address growing demand for accountability and reliable assessment tools in PA clinical practice.[9]

The first American PA competency framework, *Competencies for the Physician Assistant Profession*, emerged from a working group of the National Commission on Certification of Physician Assistants, with representation from each of the major PA organizations, known as the "Four Orgs." (The other three are the American Academy of PAs, the Physician Assistant Education Association, and the Accreditation Review Commission on Education for the Physician Assistant, Inc.) Initially, the working group considered creating a PA competency framework de novo. However, they soon realized that, owing to the strong alignment in the scope of practice of physicians and PAs, there was greater value in following the structure of the ACGME framework and adapting it to the specific features of the PA profession.

The competency framework, originally adopted in 2005 and revised in 2012, includes the same six domains found in the ACGME competency framework (although listed in a different order): (1) medical knowledge, (2) interpersonal and communication skills, (3) patient care, (4) professionalism, (5) practice-based learning and improvement, and (6) systems-based practice.[10]

CORE COMPETENCIES FOR NEW PHYSICIAN ASSISTANT GRADUATES

The original *Competencies for the Physician Assistant Profession* were developed for the purpose of providing "a foundation from which physician assistant organizations and individual physician assistants could chart a course for advancing the competencies of the PA profession." Although this was a solid foundation for PAs in practice and for the profession in general, it did not accurately reflect the competencies of newly graduating PAs.

The number of new PA programs in the United States is increasing dramatically in recent years. Since 2000, the number of PA programs accredited by the Accreditation Review Commission on Education for the Physician Assistant, Inc., has doubled from 123 to 246 in 2019.[11] Twenty-four programs were on track to become accredited between June and July of 2019 alone. A new set of competencies was created by the four Orgs to establish standards for practice readiness specifically for PA graduates. With this explosion in PA educational programs, there is an acute need for standardization of program outcomes for the profession. Although this framework was developed for entry-to-practice PAs, it may also lay a foundation for future revisions of the *Competencies for the Physician Assistant Profession*.

Beginning in 2016, led by the Physician Assistant Education Association, the four Orgs developed the *Core Competencies for New Physician Assistant Graduates (Core Competencies for New Physician Assistant Graduates).* The resulting set of six competencies mostly overlap with, but also diverge at times, from the six ACGME competency domains adopted by the Competencies for the Physician Assistant Profession. They are (1) patient-centered practice knowledge, (2) society and population health, (3) health literacy and communication, (4) interprofessional collaborative practice and leadership, (5) professional and legal aspects of healthcare, and (6) healthcare finance and systems. In addition to these six core domains, two other competency domains were applied *across* the core domains of the framework. These are (1) cultural humility and (2) self-assessment and ongoing professional development.

In the process of developing this new framework, the task force mapped and compared other healthcare professions competency frameworks with the existing PA competency framework. Some of the significant decisions included using the terminology "patient-centered practice knowledge" in place of "medical knowledge." They also emphasized quality and safety, population health, and interprofessional collaboration, across the framework.

CanMEDS PHYSICIAN ASSISTANT

The PA profession emerged in the civilian sector in Canada only in the last two decades. PAs have been working in the Canadian Armed Forces since 1984, and in similar roles for a long time before that. The first occupational competency profile was created in 2001, in collaboration with the Canadian Armed Forces and the Canadian Association of Physician Assistants. After several updates and revisions, the Canadian PA competency framework was adapted to mirror CanMEDS, first in 2009 and then in 2015, when it was renamed CanMEDS-PA.[12]

Like CanMEDS, CanMEDS-PA identifies seven thematic roles that together reflect a competent PA. In turn, a competent PA can help ensure the best patient outcomes and satisfaction with care. The seven CanMEDS-PA roles are the same as the CanMEDS roles for physicians, listed in the same order: (1) Medical Expert, (2) Communicator, (3) Collaborator, (4) Leader (manager before the 2015 update), (5) Health Advocate, (6) Scholar, and (7) Professional. Although the competency roles, are the same, the subcategories of key and enabling competencies vary according to the specific context of PA practice.

COMPARING PHYSICIAN ASSISTANT COMPETENCY FRAMEWORKS

Table 2 shows some of the similarities and differences between the competency frameworks presented previously. Notably, the competencies in the American

Table 2
Comparing three PA competency frameworks

Competency Framework	Competencies for the Physician Assistant Profession (Based on ACGME General Competencies)[10]	Core Competencies for the New PA Graduate[14]	CanMEDS-PA (Based on CanMEDS)[12]
Competencies categorizes as	Domains	Domains	Roles
Competencies	Medical knowledge	Patient-centered practice knowledge	Medical expert
	Interpersonal and communication skills	Society and population health	Communicator
	Patient care	Health literacy and communication	Collaborator
	Professionalism	Interprofessional collaborative practice and leadership	Leader
	Practice-based learning and improvement	Professional and legal aspects of healthcare	Health advocate
	Systems-based practice	Healthcare finance and systems	Scholar
			Professional

frameworks list the general categories as *domains*, whereas the Canadian frameworks use the term *roles*. The use of the term *roles* to categorize areas of competency in the Canadian frameworks for physicians and PAs dates back to the EFPO project in the late 1980s. Whitehead found "no rationale for the use of role, nor any discussion of why this approach was chosen."[13(p174)] There seems to be an implicit decision in the development of EFPO, and later CanMEDS, that identification of physician *roles* is the path to meeting societal needs. (It is interesting to note that Elam, writing in the 1970s about the teachers education movement's shift to competency-based education, asserts that competencies are "derived from explicit conceptions of teacher *roles*."[1(p15)] Could this be the origin for the use of *roles* in Canadian medical competency frameworks?)

In contrast, the term *domain* is a more general and removed categorization than *role*. A role implies embodiment of a concept and may further imply a greater responsibility to internalize the role title. The Canadian *roles* are framed as what the PA is or does (eg, medical expert, communicator, collaborator), whereas a *domain* describes attributes or values of the PA, with a bit more distance, compared with the very personalized and internalized *role* (eg, medical knowledge, interpersonal and communication skills). *Roles* can also have a negative connotation, describing a part that is played or enacted, as opposed to being authentic and real. There are many differences in the names of the *domains/roles* between the three PA competency profiles in **Table 2**. We highlight only a few here and ask the critical reader to reflect on further comparisons beyond those presented here.

Of note, all three frameworks begin with what CanMEDS considers the central competency domain: the clinical medicine knowledge base and skillset of a PA. However, the specific domain name varies by framework. It is called *medical expert*,[12] *medical knowledge*,[10] and *patient-centered practice knowledge*.[14] Medical expert is intended to highlight the distinguishing, central feature of a PA from a ley person. Although nonmedical professionals may have expertise in the supporting, relational roles of

CanMEDS-PA, the PA is an expert in medicine. *Patient-centered practice knowledge* differs from *medical expert* and *medical knowledge* by emphasizing the centrality of the patient in the application of medical knowledge.

The Canadian and American healthcare systems vary in their structure and function, a topic that has been highlighted in the media and political conversation in recent years. Canada has long embraced the concept of universal publicly funded, single-payer healthcare coverage, commonly referred to as Medicare. In contrast, the United States continues a long debate about public versus private funding of healthcare services. Some services for disadvantaged or other populations are covered by government programs in the U.S. (eg, Medicare and Medicaid). Others may be covered by private insurance, either paid for out of pocket or by employment benefits. The large proportion of uninsured people and often prohibitive healthcare costs in the United States is a major social and financial burden. In general, with the multipayer US system and many different insurance companies, the American healthcare system is more complex and challenging to navigate. It makes sense, then, that the two American frameworks, but not the Canadian framework, have a competency domain specifically related to navigating the healthcare system: *systems-based practice*[14] and *healthcare finance and systems.*[14]

BEYOND COMPETENCY FRAMEWORKS

The challenge that emerged after the development of the first competency frameworks was the gap between theory and implementation of CBME. Program leaders and faculty members struggled to understand what the competencies meant, what they looked like in day-to-day practice, and how to objectively measure them. These challenges especially applied to competencies that did not readily lend themselves to observation or objective measurement, such as professionalism or health advocacy. Another challenge that emerged related to the learning continuum itself. Competence can not be static along the learning trajectory—expectations for an early learner should not be the same as expectations for a more advanced learner, or for someone ready to enter clinical practice. How can CBME account for these varying benchmarks along the learning journey?

The practical need to interpret and operationalize the competency frameworks gave rise to a number of new initiatives to help implement CBME in the past decade or so. These include Milestones, EPA, and Competence by Design, which are described here.

MILESTONES

In 2009, the ACMGE launched the Milestones project as a part of the Next Accreditation System to advance the utility of the Outcomes Project and the General Competencies. Milestones were designed to provide narrative descriptions of the competencies and subcompetencies in the ACGME competency framework. Essentially, Milestones are anchors that describe where a learner is situated along the developmental continuum, for each specific subcompetency. The continuum is modeled according to the 5-stage Dreyfus model of expertise[15] and describes the expected level for a new resident (novice), before mid-residency (advanced beginner), at mid-residency (competence), at the end of residency (proficiency), and beyond these expectations (expertise) as shown in the Milestones template in **Fig. 2**. Milestones can be used for the assessment of learner performance at various levels of development, both for summative and formative feedback. Milestones can also be used as a shared language or mental model among residency programs and as a national standard within a specialty (**Fig. 2**). An example of Milestones for a specific subcompetency under the medical knowledge domain can be seen in **Fig. 3**.

ENTRUSTABLE PROFESSIONAL ACTIVITIES

The concept of EPAs was first proposed in 2005 as a means to bridge the gap between the theories of CBME and the day-to-day practice of clinical work.[16] Olle ten Cate, a Dutch medical educator, recognized that, although CBME had gained wide and rapid popularity in the previous decade, it was now at risk of "competencies hype" and could fade into memory as "essentially nothing but a label, replacing what we conveniently used to call 'educational objectives.'"[16(p1176)] Similar to Milestones, EPAs do not replace competency-based education; rather, they offer a bridge between the potentially overly deconstructed and context-free elements of competencies and the realities of daily clinical work. EPAs can be viewed as an evolution from CBME, rather than an entirely new entity.

EPAs are defined as "units of work." They shift the focus away from the ability of the learner and toward the clinical task or activity. The relevant question is whether the trainee can be entrusted to perform this task or activity without direct supervision.

An EPA is a work-based activity that may include a number of individual competencies. Visual representations of EPAs illustrate the relationship between EPAs and competencies by using a grid of EPAs along one side and competency domains along the other. For example, an EPA such as "discussing medical errors with patients" would include competence in the domains of interpersonal skills and communication, professionalism, practice-based learning and improvement, and systems-based practice. Another EPA, such as initiating cardiopulmonary resuscitation, would include competence in medical knowledge and patient care.[17]

An interesting historical link between EPAs and PA education is worth noting. The University of Applied Science in Utrecht, the Netherlands, used EPAs to develop the clinical training for their PA program.[18] **Table 3**, taken from a neurology PA educational curriculum at The University of Applied Science, demonstrates the relationships

General Description of Milestone Levels

Milestone Description: Template				
Level 1	Level 2	Level 3	Level 4	Level 5
What are the expectations for a beginning resident?	What are the milestones for a resident who has advanced over entry, but is performing at a lower level than expected at mid-residency?	What are the key developmental milestones mid-residency? What should they be able to do well in the realm of the specialty at this point?	What does a graduating resident look like? What additional knowledge, skills & attitudes have they obtained? Are they ready for certification?	Stretch Goals – Exceeds expectations
☐ ☐ ☐ ☐ ☐ ☐ ☐ ☐ ☐				
Comments:				

Fig. 2. General description of milestone levels. (*From* Holmboe ES, Edgar L, Hamstra SJ. The Milestones Guidebook. Chicago, IL: Accreditation Council for Graduate Medical Education; 2016. Available at: http://www.acgme.org/Portals/0/MilestonesGuidebook.pdf?ver=2016-05-31-113245-103; with permission.)

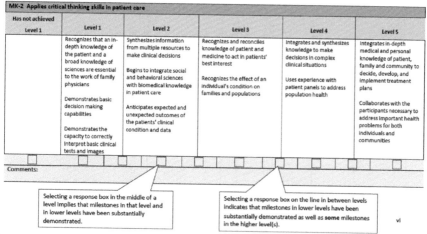

Fig. 3. Milestones for specific sub competency. (*From* The family medicine milestone project. J Grad Med Educ. 2014 Mar;6(1 Suppl 1):74-86. https://doi.org/10.4300/JGME-06-01s1-05; with permission.)

between the five identified EPAs for this clinical curriculum and the seven competency domains.

Looking at the third EPA as an example, "Care for the stroke patients" (see **Table 3**); this EPA encompasses the domains of communication, collaboration, health advocacy, and professionalism. Each of the EPAs is further elaborated and described, as in the example used in **Table 4**. For each of the EPAs in the clinical training, a learner is expected to achieve progressive degrees of entrustability and decreasing requirements for direct supervision through the course of training. For the cited example, the learner should be able to perform these activities under full supervision only in the second block of training (a block is approximately 10 weeks), with limited supervision in blocks three to five, and with back stage supervision by block six.[18]

Many medical educational programs are incorporating EPAs in their curricula. Canadian PA education is also considering updating curricular and accreditation standards to reflect EPAs for PAs.[19]

COMPETENCE BY DESIGN

In 2017, The Royal College of Physicians and Surgeons of Canada launched their Competence by Design (CBD) project with the first two medical specialties adopting CBD into their curriculum—otolaryngology–head and neck surgery and anesthesiology.[20] CBD focuses on the developmental stages of resident education and establishes specific outcomes for teaching and learning along this continuum. CBD incorporates both Milestones and EPAs.

There are four developmental stages identified by CBD that span from entry to residency to entry to practice: (1) *transition to discipline* focuses on the orientation of the new resident, sometimes referred to as the junior resident, (2) *foundations of discipline* refers to basic general competencies common for all residents, (3) *core of discipline* covers more advanced, discipline-specific competencies, and (4) *transition to practice,* when the resident is deemed ready for independent practice.[21]

Table 3
The 5 EPAs

	Medical Expertise	Communication	Collaboration	Scholarship	Health Advocacy	Management	Professionalism
1 Taking first history and physical of neurology patients	X	X	—	—	—	X	X
2 Performing lumbar punctures	X	—	X	—	—	X	—
3 Care for stroke patients	—	X	X	—	X	—	X
4 Care for patients with lumbosacral radicular complaints	—	X	X	—	X	X	X
5 Care for patients with a carpal tunnel syndrome (CTS)	X	X	X	X	—	X	—

From Mulder H, Cate OT, Daalder R, et al. Building a competency-based workplace curriculum around entrustable professional activities: The case of physician assistant training. Medical Teacher, 32(10), e453-e459. https://doi.org/10.3109/0142159X.2010.513719; with permission.

Table 4	
Descriptions of EPA use	
Discipline	**Neurology**
Title of the EPA	Care for stroke patients
Short description	Care for noncomplicated stroke patients after initial diagnosis until release from the hospital, including selecting, requesting and interpreting diagnostic tests and taking subsequent measures; recognition of complications; communicating with family and colleagues; chairing focused multidisciplinary meetings; and handling correspondence with the patient's family doctor
Occurrence frequency	One or more times per day
Most important CanMEDS domains of competence	Communication, collaboration, health advocacy, professionalism
Knowledge and skills required	Knowledge of neuroanatomy, including vascularization areas Knowledge of pathology related to stroke symptoms: TIA, bleeding CVA, ischemic CVA, insult Knowledge and management skills concerning common complications: pneumonia, UG infection Knowledge and skill to interpret diagnostic tests: CT scan, duplex, MRI, MRA, laboratory tests, ECG Knowledge of medication policy with hospitalized patients with stroke symptoms Knowledge of secondary prevention measures of patient hospitalized for stroke Knowledge and skill to deal with the local healthcare organization and rules Knowledge of contraindicated treatments for hospitalized stoke patients Ability to do a focused history and physical examination skills, including investigating consciousness, cranial nerves, locomotion, sensibility, reflexes, and coordination Ability to chair multidisciplinary meetings Ability to communicate well with family other healthcare workers about diagnosis, treatment, prognosis and secondary prevention
Assessment procedure	Detailed observation or shadowing of the whole process a number of times Structured interviewing about procedural knowledge

Abbreviations: CT, computed tomography; CVA, cerebrovascular accident; ECG, electrocardiogram; EPA, entrustable professional activity; MRA, magnetic resonance angiography; TIA, transient ischemic attack.

From Mulder H, Cate OT, Daalder R, et al. Building a competency-based workplace curriculum around entrustable professional activities: The case of physician assistant training. Medical Teacher, 32(10), e453-e459. https://doi.org/10.3109/0142159X.2010.513719; with permission.

CRITIQUE OF COMPETENCY FRAMEWORKS

CBME has generally been accepted as an effective framework for medical curricula for the purposes of teaching, learning, assessment, certification, and accreditation. CBME and the various associated competency frameworks have indeed revolutionized healthcare education. CBME has introduced many improvements in how physicians, PAs, and other healthcare professionals are educated and practice. These improvements include better standardization and objectivity in education and assessment. Perhaps most important, competency frameworks have identified and assigned value to abilities beyond the knowledge of pathophysiology or technical skills; that is, the relational competency domains, such as communication and collaboration.

It makes sense that a framework of specific observable abilities and attributes is a practical tool to contain this vast compliment of knowledge, skills, and attitudes. This is especially true at a time of rapid expansion in medical knowledge and technological advances; a public demanding transparency and with access to troves of healthcare information; a more complex, integrated healthcare system; and increasing specialization.

However, CBME, which gained wide popularity globally in the late twentieth century, and is still going strong, does have its critics and skeptics.[22–24] Some of the reasons for the criticism of CBME relate to its checklist-oriented nature; the questionable notion of objectivity in observing and assessing acquisition of competence; the loss of integration between individual, deconstructed components of competence; the lack of real-world clinical context in their attainment and assessment; and the potential interference with professional identity formation. As with any novel trend or fashion, there is a risk of overemphasizing certain values at the expense of others. CBME is no exception, and some significant criticism has emerged.

Competence in the discourse of health professions education and practice in recent decades has been called a "god term."[25] Lingard uses this expression, coined earlier by the literary critic Kenneth Burke, to identify the word *competency* as a "rhetorical trump card."[25(p625)] She suggests that the focus on competence in its current use in the health professions overemphasizes the health professional's individual abilities. The learner's or clinician's competence is assessed and determined outside the context in which it is to be applied—that is, the real-world, uncertain, and ever-changing clinical context. Furthermore, Lingard suggests that competency-based education and practice ignore theories of social learning that better account for learning and applying knowledge in real-world context. She illustrates this most clearly by describing how "competent individual professionals can—and do, with some regularity—combine to create an incompetent team."[25(p626)]

What we choose to focus on when we identify a competent PA may also have unwanted side effects based on what that particular discourse excludes.[26] Hodges describes several current discourses of competence that emphasize specific elements, and by doing so, may neglect others. His examples include discourses that characterize competence in various ways, such as competence as knowledge, competence as performance, competence as reliable test scores, and competence as reflection. In each of these examples, it is important to consider the benefits and drawbacks of emphasizing or overemphasizing one value over others.

Hodges[26] argues that, of themselves, none of these discourses is wrong or wholly inappropriate, but that the thoughtful health professional and educator should pay attention to what is emphasized and what is minimized. This deliberate focus on the power of discourse will help avoid developing incompetence in some areas while, with the best intentions, we develop competence in other areas.

Another critique of the current shift to a competency-based model of education and practice is the implied conclusion that healthcare professionals are ready to practice when they have demonstrated competence in the required areas. Not only are these discrete demonstrations of individual competence disembodied from the context of their application, as described elsewhere in this article, but this approach also ignores the socialization and acculturation of a novice into the health profession. Development of professional identity is arguably as important as acquisition of discrete abilities.[27,28]

Professional identity formation is considered "an active, developmental process which is dynamic and constructive and is an essential complement to competency-based education."[29(p701)]

Hodges refers to the older traditional methods of medical education as "tea-steeping"—a process in which the novice medical learner is placed into the environment of medical school. Just as a teabag sitting in hot water for a fixed period of time results in a cup of tea, the medical student, after absorbing the educational content and cultural milieu in medical school for a fixed period of time, presumably becomes a physician.[30] This more passive-sounding approach contrasts with CBME, in which the learner must be a more active participant in the learning progression, continually demonstrating attainment of competence. Although tea-steeping may describe the traditional time-based medical curricula in an uncomplimentary light, compared with CBME, it does reflect a perhaps desirable element of immersive learning—a nod to identity formation through exposure and acculturation to a profession.

One final critique of competency-based education and practice is the "missing person" in the roles-based frameworks.[31] During the development of the RCPSC's Can-MEDS framework, an eighth role that was considered but ultimately omitted as a role in its own right was that of *person* (as in, physician as person). Whitehead and colleagues[31] explain that the names of the roles in the CanMEDS framework should not be considered self-evident or naturally occurring, but rather developed in a specific historical and cultural context. (In the Netherlands, at the VU University Medical Center, the role of reflector was added as an eighth role to the curriculum. Similarly, the University of Ottawa's medical program retained the person role in their ePortfolio program.[32])

In examining the contrast between CanMEDS, which chose to incorporate the concepts of physician identify and wellness in the Professional Role, and examples of educational frameworks that added a reflector role, Whitehead and colleagues[31] consider the purpose of the roles in the first place. In a framework that deemphasizes the physician as a person, greater emphasis seems to be on societal demands of physicians, whereas frameworks that include person or reflector roles seem to assign more value to the individual development and personal well-being of the medical learner and practitioner.

SUMMARY

CBME and competency frameworks, introduced in the 1990s, are arguably the greatest contributions to the renewal of medical education since Abraham Flexner revolutionized the field with his Flexner Report in 1910. The benefits of CBME include clear identification of learning outcomes to guide teaching and assessment; the ability to standardize curricula across jurisdictions and institutions, and establish criteria for accreditation, certification, and licensure; and the identification of interpersonal and professional skills that were previously undervalued compared with clinical knowledge and technical skills.

Although professional competency frameworks for physicians, PAs, and other professions have established criteria for a competent healthcare professional, the gap between the theory of these frameworks and their application to the real-world clinical setting has been a challenge for educators. Several complimentary approaches, such as Milestones, EPAs, and Competence by Design, have been developed to bridge this gap and facilitate the implementation of CBME.

Although generally successful and popular, CBME has been criticized as overly deconstructive, missing the big picture by overemphasizing its granular components.

Other criticisms include the loss of focus on the health professional's identity and personhood, and the focus on competence as a god-term, or a discursive trump card. By considering and addressing the strengths and pitfalls of CBME, and by comparing various competency frameworks to highlight meaningful similarities and differences, PA educators and practicing PAs can continue to refine and strengthen these valuable tools.

ACKNOWLEDGMENTS

The author would like to thank the Consortium of PA Education, the Department of Family & Community Medicine, and the University of Toronto for supporting the preparation of this article.

REFERENCES

1. Elam S. Performance-based teacher education: what is the state of the art? Quest 1972;18(1):14–9.
2. Carraccio CMD, Wolfsthal SDMD, Englander R, et al. Shifting paradigms: from Flexner to competencies. Acad Med 2002;77(5):361–7.
3. Curry L, Wergin JF. Educating professionals: responding to new expectations for competence and accountability. San Francisco (CA): Jossey-Bass; 1993.
4. Kizer KW. Establishing health care performance standards in an era of consumerism. JAMA 2001;286(10):1213–7.
5. Lanier DC, Roland M, Burstin H, et al. Doctor performance and public accountability. Lancet 2003;362(9393):1404–8.
6. Swing SR. The ACGME outcome project: retrospective and prospective. Med Teach 2007;29(7):648–54.
7. Butt H, Duffin J. Educating future physicians for Ontario and the physicians' strike of 1986: the roots of Canadian competency-based medical education. CMAJ 2018;190(7):E196–8.
8. Educating Future Physicians for Ontario Project. What people of Ontario need and expect from physicians. Hamilton, Ontario: EFPO Co-ordinating Centre; 1993.
9. Competencies for the physician assistant profession. JAAPA 2005;18(7):16–8.
10. Competencies for the physician assistant profession. 2012. Available at: https://prodcmsstoragesa.blob.core.windows.net/uploads/files/PACompetencies.pdf. Accessed August 22, 2019.
11. Accreditation Review Commission on Education for the Physician Assistant. Available at: http://www.arc-pa.org/wp-content/uploads/2019/07/Accred-Prog-Graph-thru-6.2019.pdf.
12. Canadian Association for Physician Assistants. CanMEDS-PA. Available at: https://capa-acam.ca/wp-content/uploads/2015/11/CanMEDS-PA.pdf
13. Whitehead C. The good doctor in medical education 1910–2010: a critical discourse analysis. Ann Arbor (MI): University of Toronto (Canada); 2011. Dissertations & Theses @ University of Toronto; ProQuest Dissertations & Theses Global database. (NR79370). Available at: https://search-proquest-com.myaccess.library.utoronto.ca/docview/1325198992#.
14. Physician Assistant Education Association. Core Competencies for New Physician Assistant Graduates. Available at: https://paeaonline.org/wp-content/uploads/2018/09/core-competencies-for-pa-grads-20180919.pdf. Accessed October 25, 2018.

15. Dreyfus SE. The Five-Stage Model of Adult Skill Acquisition. Bulletin of Science, Technology & Society 2004;24(3):177–81.
16. ten Cate O. Entrustability of professional activities and competency-based training. Med Educ 2005;39(12):1176–7.
17. ten Cate O. AM last page: what entrustable professional activities add to a competency-based curriculum. Acad Med 2014;89(4):691.
18. Mulder H, ten Cate O, Daalder R, et al. Building a competency-based workplace curriculum around entrustable professional activities: the case of physician assistant training. Med Teach 2010;32(10):e453–9.
19. Burrows KE, Jones IW. 2018 Annual conference of the Canadian Assoication of Physician Assistants. Available at: https://capa-acam.ca/faqs/cpaea-poster-presentations/.
20. Competence by Design: making medical education history. (2017). Competence by Design. Available at: http://www.royalcollege.ca/rcsite/cbd/cbd-launch-medical-education-history-e. Accessed August 15, 2019.
21. CBD competence continuum. Ottawa (Canada): Royal College of Physicians and Surgeons of Canada; 2015.
22. Brooks MA. Medical education and the tyranny of competency. Perspect Biol Med 2009;52(1):90–102.
23. Whitehead C, Austin Z, Hodges B. Flower power: the armoured expert in the CanMEDS competency framework? Adv Health Sci Educ Theory Pract 2011;16(5):681–94.
24. Whitehead CR, Kuper A. Faith-based medical education. Adv Health Sci Educ Theory Pract 2017;22(1):1–3.
25. Lingard L. What we see and don't see when we look at 'competence': notes on a god term. Adv Health Sci Educ Theory Pract 2009;14(5):625–8.
26. Hodges B. Medical Education and the Maintenance of Incompetence. Medical Teacher 2006;28(8):690–6.
27. Cruess RL, Cruess SR, Boudreau JD, et al. Reframing Medical Education to Support Professional Identity Formation. Acad Med 2014;89(11):1446–51.
28. Jarvis-Selinger S, Pratt DD, Regehr G. Competency Is Not Enough. Academic Medicine 2012;87(9):1185–90.
29. Wald HSP. Professional identity (trans)formation in medical education: reflection, relationship, resilience. Acad Med 2015;90(6):701–6.
30. Hodges BD. A Tea-Steeping or i-Doc Model for Medical Education? [Miscellaneous]. Acad Med 2010;85(9 Suppl):S134–44.
31. Whitehead C, Selleger V, van de Kreeke J, et al. The 'missing person' in roles-based competency models: a historical, cross-national, contrastive case study. Med Educ 2014;48(8):785–95.
32. University of Ottawa Faculty of Medicine ePortfolio. Available at: https://www.med.uottawa.ca/ePortfolio/. Accessed April 30, 2019.

Moving?

Make sure your subscription moves with you!

To notify us of your new address, find your **Clinics Account Number** (located on your mailing label above your name), and contact customer service at:

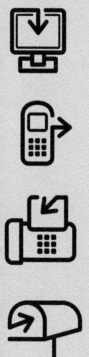

Email: journalscustomerservice-usa@elsevier.com

800-654-2452 (subscribers in the U.S. & Canada)
314-447-8871 (subscribers outside of the U.S. & Canada)

Fax number: 314-447-8029

Elsevier Health Sciences Division
Subscription Customer Service
3251 Riverport Lane
Maryland Heights, MO 63043